EARL MINDELL'S

Arthritis

EARL MINDELL'S

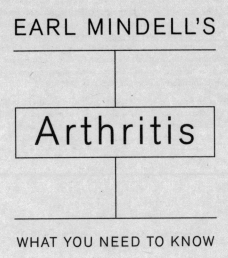

Arthritis

WHAT YOU NEED TO KNOW

Earl Mindell, R.Ph., Ph.D.,
and Melissa Block, M.Ed.

AVERY
a member of Penguin Putnam Inc.
NEW YORK

Most Avery books are available at special quantity discounts for bulk purchase for sales promotions, premiums, fund-raising, and educational needs. Special books or book excerpts also can be created to fit specific needs. For details, write Putnam Special Markets, 375 Hudson Street, New York, NY 10014.

Avery
a member of
Penguin Putnam Inc.
375 Hudson Street
New York, NY 10014
www.penguinputnam.com

Library of Congress Cataloging-in-Publication Data

Mindell, Earl.
[Arthritis]
Earl Mindell's arthritis : What you need to know / Earl Mindell &
Melissa Block.
p.   cm.
Includes bibliographical references and index.
ISBN 1-58333-081-X
1. Arthritis—Popular works.   2. Arthritis—Treatment—Popular
works.   3. Consumer education.   I. Block, Melissa.   II. Title.
III. Series.

RC933 .M56   2000   00-042016
616.7'22—dc21

Printed in the United States of America

1   3   5   7   9   10   8   6   4   2

Book design by Jennifer Ann Daddio
Cover design by Jess Morphew

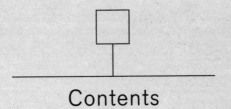

Contents

EARL MINDELL'S

Arthritis

1

Ten Core Principles
for Healthy Living

In this book, you'll learn everything you ever wanted to know about arthritis. You'll learn what the typical conventional treatments are, and about any potential health hazards you may encounter as a result of those treatments. You'll learn about safe, effective natural remedies that work synergistically with your body's natural tendency toward healing and balance, rather than against them. The right natural remedies for arthritis can keep you off prescription drugs and out of the hospital. No natural remedy, however, is going to heal your body if you aren't doing all you can to bring it to a state of general good health.

The Ten Core Principles for Healthy Living are your guide for taking excellent care of yourself and embracing a healthy lifestyle. It's as simple as following these ten guidelines, which I have developed over more than thirty years of research, lecturing, and writing. Whether you implement only one or two of them or make a major lifestyle overhaul, these ten principles will work together or separately to improve your health.

1.
Eat Whole Foods
Instead of Processed Foods

Chronic diseases such as heart disease, diabetes, cancer, arthritis, osteoporosis, allergies, asthma, and autoimmune disease are affecting more people in modernized nations than ever before. The medical research community has put much effort into pinpointing the causes of these diseases. They've come up with a wide variety of possible causes: genetic predisposition, too much fat in the diet, certain kinds of fat in the diet, certain chemicals in the environment, viruses, too much sugar, not enough calcium, and countless others. If you're trying your best to prevent or heal chronic disease, you may often find yourself confused by conflicting advice based on the latest theories.

I believe one of the most important answers to this state of affairs is a simple one: that a diet of refined, processed foods, rather than fresh, whole foods, plays a major role in the increase in chronic diseases. Refined and processed foods include canned and frozen food, refined white flour products (breads, bagels, baked goods, pasta), chips, sweets, meats such as bologna and hot dogs, and all the rest of those foods lining the grocery store shelves that are long on sugary, salty, or fatty taste and short on nutrition.

Refinement and processing of foods strips them of their nutritional value. Refined foods tend to have strong, even addictive tastes compared to vegetables, fruits, and whole grains, but they are appetizing only because of all the sugar, salt, oils, and other additives and flavorings they contain. Food manufacturers sometimes add vitamins and minerals to their products, but this hardly makes them equal in nutritional value to whole foods.

Whole foods are those that have undergone minimal or no processing, that are as close as possible to their natural state. The staples of a whole-foods diet are fresh vegetables, whole grains, legumes (beans), fruit, raw nuts and seeds, and occasional servings of organic meats, fish, poultry, and dairy products. Herbs, spices, and healthy oils add flavor and variety. (More diet specifics will be given later in the book.)

Contrary to popular belief, this kind of diet can be delicious and satisfying. Our taste buds have grown accustomed to the powerful and addictive tastes of sugar, salt, and other artificial flavorings. Whole foods have more delicate flavors that we need to adjust to if we've been eating primarily refined foods. Once you make the shift, though, you'll feel so much better that you'll never want to go back.

A whole-foods diet is one of the surest ways to keep your body youthful, energetic, slim, and free of disease. Of course, it's hard for some people to imagine eating nothing but whole foods. Even if you can't go all the way with it, try to replace processed foods with whole foods whenever you can. There are a few non-negotiables here, however.

Kick your sugar habit. Americans eat approximately 133 pounds of sugar a year. Sugar—including white and brown varieties, fructose (fruit sugar), maple syrup, and honey—all cause blood sugar levels to fluctuate. When you eat a sugary snack, your blood sugar rises way above normal. High blood sugar is harmful to the body in many ways, and so the pancreas comes to the rescue, pumping out plenty of insulin. Insulin's job is to pull sugar out of the blood and store it in the cells. It does its job so well that blood sugar levels plummet. You then suffer from the shakes, foggy thinking, and fatigue, and soon you're craving another dose of refined sugar.

Sugar depletes your body of B vitamins and the minerals magnesium, chromium, and copper. It suppresses your immune system, damages your kidneys, worsens allergies, and raises blood fats (cholesterol and triglycerides). It's true that some forms of sugar are less harmful than others—honey and maple sugar are less refined, and so have a less intense effect—but they'll put you on the sugar-addiction treadmill just as the others do. Your best bet is to break your sugar habit entirely and to reserve sweets for the most special of occasions.

Bypass the bread and pass on the pasta. When the medical community began to recommend a low-fat diet for weight loss and prevention of disease, throngs of health-minded people took notice. Rather than eating more vegetables and fruits, which are naturally low in fat, many turned to processed, packaged "low-fat" snacks and staples: pasta, pretzels, bread, and sugary snacks. Consumers were blitzed with advertising implying that if a food was low in fat, it was healthy. What they weren't told was that flour—especially white flour—has virtually the same effect on the body as sugar does. When wheat is stripped of its husk and oils and made into flour, it's called an unrefined carbohydrate and it essentially becomes sugar. It has virtually no nutritional value and causes blood sugar to swing rapidly up and down. Making these foods your mainstay is only slightly healthier than living on sweets.

If you can't live without bread, find a variety made with the whole grain. They should say "whole grain" on the label, not just "whole wheat." Corn tortillas are another healthful alternative to bread. Use whole grains—

brown rice, quinoa, barley, polenta, and millet—instead of pasta. They cook up quickly and taste great with vegetables.

Use healthy oils. Recent research has revealed that the *amount* of fat you eat is less important than the *type* of fat you eat. There are three major categories of fats that exist in whole foods: saturated (found in meats and dairy products), monounsaturated (found in olive, canola, and avocado oils), and polyunsaturated (found in nut, seed, and soybean oils).

The saturation of a fat molecule describes the stability of that fat—its resistance to spoiling, or *oxidizing.* Oxidation is a natural process that occurs when fats are exposed to oxygen, creating free radicals, which damage cells. The more saturated the fat, the more resistant it is to oxidation.

The body uses antioxidant nutrients, such as vitamins C and E, to neutralize free radicals. If our free radical load is high and our antioxidant intake low, the overflow of oxidation can be highly destructive to our tissues. Excess free radicals are a likely common denominator in the causes of many chronic diseases, especially cancer and heart disease.

Saturated fats have been blamed for everything from heart disease to cancer, but they are only dangerous in excess. A small amount of butter or whole milk adds a lot of flavor to foods, and if you add these fats to your diet in moderate amounts they shouldn't cause you any harm. Polyunsaturated fats, and their close cousins, the hydrogenated fats, are the ones to avoid. Polyunsaturated fats, such as corn oil, safflower oil, and cottonseed oil, are very unstable and oxidize easily. Heating them to high temperatures for cooking produces many free radicals.

Hydrogenated oils are the food industry's attempt to solve this problem. By bombarding unsaturated oils with hydrogen atoms, food manufacturers create fats that are more stable and resistant to spoilage. It turns out, however, that these fake fats contain trans-fatty acids that increase the risk of artery-clogging plaques and heart attacks. They are much worse for you than any saturated oil, and not much better than the rancid unsaturated oils. Virtually all processed and refined foods contain hydrogenated or "partially hydrogenated" oils.

The gold standard is monounsaturated oil. Olive oil is your best bet; it's delicious, and the extra virgin varieties are only minimally processed. Canola oil is best for baking and cooking foods that don't taste right with olive oil. These oils are only slightly less stable than saturated fats. The olive oil–rich Mediterranean diet has been shown to reduce risk of heart disease.

Eat your fish. Deepwater fish, such as salmon, mackerel, and cod, are loaded with heart-healthy omega-3 fats. These fats are polyunsaturated, but in their natural form (fish) they do not go rancid before the fish goes bad, and they have potent anti-inflammatory effects, lower cholesterol, protect against certain forms of cancer, and help to thin the blood (which helps prevent blood clots that cause heart attacks and strokes). Enjoy baked or poached fish two or three times a week.

Make raw foods a part of your daily diet. Raw foods contain enzymes that aid digestion and absorption of nutrients. Most people eat virtually no raw food. Cooking shuts off all enzyme activity and destroys water-soluble vitamins such as vitamin C. Fresh fruit at breakfast and a green salad with dinner are excellent ways to add raw foods to your diet. Buy locally grown produce whenever you can; when it sits for long periods in trucks and on supermarket shelves, levels of enzymes and vitamins decrease.

2.
Drink Plenty of Clean Water Every Day

Your body is two-thirds water. Think of that water as a crystal clear mountain lake. Now imagine that lake becoming stagnant because the streams that bring water into and out of it stop flowing. A stagnant lake becomes clouded and overgrown with algae. Now, imagine a campground being built next to the lake, bringing with it trash and sewage. More and more toxins come in, and there is no moving fresh water to flush them away. Eventually, the lake becomes uninhabitable to the life forms that once thrived there.

This is what happens in your body when you eat what we've come to call the Standard American Diet (SAD), which consists of processed foods high in sugar and fat, and when you don't drink enough water. If you don't constantly flush toxins from the water that makes up much of your body, they build up and can cause chronic disease. Even if you eat a whole-foods diet, you're still exposed to plenty of environmental toxins.

Drinking six to eight eight-ounce glasses of pure water a day—not coffee, not juice, not milk, but water—is one of the simplest things you can do to improve your health. The results will be apparent within a few days. Your skin will glow, your bowels will move more regularly, and it will be easier to control your weight. In many cases, blood cholesterol levels drop. If you down your first glass or two when you get up in the morning, you'll find yourself becoming alert and awake without caffeine. If you keep a pitcher of water with lemon slices in your refrigerator, you'll always have a cold, delicious beverage handy when you want it.

Tap water simply isn't safe to drink. Depending on where you live and where your water comes from, the types of toxins that flow from your tap will vary. Heavy metals, benzene, chlorine, and carcinogenic agricultural chemicals are typical findings in tap water. Bottled water is expensive, and its quality isn't always assured. Anyone serious about improving their health should buy a water filtration system. You can buy them for a single tap or for your whole house. The best types of filters are reverse osmosis, distillation, and ceramic; the latter is the least expensive of the three.

3.
Go Organic

When you sit down to a meal, you don't intend to eat polychlorinated biphenyls, phthalates, bovine growth hormones, altered fruit and vegetable genes, organochlorine pesticides, antibiotics, or insecticides. If you aren't eating organic produce, grains, meats, eggs, and dairy products, it's a safe bet these toxins are a part of your daily diet. If you're eating processed foods, you're probably swallowing monosodium glutamate (MSG), aspartame, tartrazine, sodium benzoate, sodium nitrite, and a host of other additives and preservatives with your meals.

The chemicals listed above have been linked with a wide variety of chronic diseases, including cancer, liver disease, brain disease, autoimmune diseases, and diseases of the reproductive tract. Despite the food and chemical industries' efforts to minimize public knowledge of the harm these toxic substances can do, more people than ever before are taking the initiative to find out the truth—and they're buying organic.

Most cattle and poultry in North America are raised in

crowded conditions and fed a diet that is far from optimal. As a result, they are riddled with diseases for which they are fed antibiotics and other drugs. Before they are sent to market they are fed estrogens to fatten them up. Those drugs end up in your body when you eat their meat or eggs or drink their milk. Vegetables, fruits, and grains that are not organic are sprayed with pesticides, fungicides, chemical fertilizers, weed killers, and petrochemical-containing waxes.

The companies that make these chemicals insist that they are safe in the amounts people are exposed to. They said that about DDT, asbestos, and atrazine, too—chemicals that were finally banned when the evidence became overwhelming that they were carcinogenic and hormone-altering. When a new chemical is introduced, it goes through basic animal testing to be sure it doesn't cause birth defects or cancer. What we know now, however, is that often the harmful effects of chemical toxins don't appear until years after being exposed, or in the offspring of people or animals who have been exposed. Until there is overwhelming evidence of an approved chemical's toxicity, it can stay on the market. The evidence that chemical toxins that are used on crops are harming humans, animals, and the environment continues to grow. The interactions between different chemicals are impossible to predict, and the typical person is exposed to dozens of different ones a day, in various combinations. Your best bet is to avoid them whenever you can. Eating organic food is one way to accomplish this end.

Organic foods are raised and grown under strict guidelines. Only natural methods are used on crops to get rid of pests and to encourage plants to grow. Animals raised organically are kept in humane conditions and are fed only organic feed. Organics are more expensive, because the process of raising them is more labor-intensive, but they're definitely worth it. The number of food dollars being spent on organics has already made conventional farmers take notice: they recently tried to persuade the government to make the guidelines much more lenient. Rather than changing their mode of operations, the industry attempted to change the rules so that their present chemical-intensive practices would be considered organic! Fortunately, well-informed consumers made such an uproar about these proposed changes that they didn't go into effect.

If you only switch one part of your diet to organics, make it animal foods—meat, poultry, dairy, and eggs. Some of the most dangerous toxins become concentrated in the fat of animal foods, and that's where you get the highest doses of these chemicals. One exception to this rule is fish, for which a set of organic labeling requirements hasn't been made. Eat more of the deep-water varieties such as salmon, cod, sardines, and mackerel. Tuna and swordfish have a higher level of mercury than most fish, so don't eat them more than once a week. Generally avoid bottom-feeding shellfish such as clams and oysters.

Conventional cleaning supplies, bug sprays, air fresheners, and beauty products also contain many ingredients with unknown or harmful effects on the body. It isn't necessary to find "organic" products for these purposes, but finding natural alternatives in your health food store will lower your toxic load substantially. You can also make your own cleaning supplies and insect repellents from natural ingredients. More nontoxic choices are available, now that people are becoming aware of the threat of living and working in a soup of chemical fumes.

4.
Support Your Digestive System

If your digestive system isn't in good working condition, eating well and taking supplements isn't going to do you a lot of good. A healthy stomach and small intestines thoroughly break food down into proteins, carbohydrates, fats, vitamins, and minerals, and absorb them into the bloodstream. The small intestines also provide a highly selective barrier designed not to allow anything potentially toxic to pass into the circulation. A healthy large intestine maintains the proper balance of water and minerals in the body and provides a home for friendly bacteria, or probiotics. Probiotics make important vitamins and keep less friendly bacteria and yeasts, which occur naturally in the body, from becoming overgrown and causing illness.

Many of the chronic illnesses that are becoming so common—including irritable bowel syndrome, arthritis, asthma, allergies, chronic fatigue syndrome, depression, and autoimmune disease—can be traced back to imbalances in the digestive system. These imbalances are directly related to the consumption of the processed-food, nutrient-depleted SAD. Conventional medicine has not yet recognized the importance of a balanced digestive system, making the above diseases difficult for conventional doctors to diagnose or treat.

Digestive problems can begin in the stomach, small intestines, or large intestines. These organs are interdependent, and as soon as one weakens, the others are compromised. A large proportion of people make insufficient stomach acid to break food down thoroughly. This is especially likely for people who suffer from heartburn or feelings of fullness for hours after eating.

You can support your digestive function with the right diet, but if you've been eating the SAD for some time, or if you have chronic indigestion or irritable bowel syndrome, you'll need a little extra help to get back on track. Try taking a digestive enzyme and betaine HCl (hydrochloric acid) supplement at each meal. Make sure it contains protein, fat, and carbohydrate-digesting enzymes—protease, lipase, and amylase, respectively. To ensure that you have adequate friendly bacteria, keep a refrigerated probiotic supplement on hand, and take it between meals, especially if you have recently had to use antibiotics. Antibiotics indiscriminately kill off good and bad bacteria.

It's also important to get plenty of fiber in your diet, which you will do if you're eating the whole-foods diet in step 1. Fiber is found in unprocessed fruits and vegetables, whole grains, nuts, and seeds.

If you follow the diet guidelines and use these digestive supplements as needed, you'll get the very most out of your food.

5.
Vitamin and Mineral Supplements: The Best Health Insurance

If you are committed to enjoying optimal health, be prepared to add nutritional supplements to your whole-foods diet. Vitamin and mineral supplements ensure that your body never lacks the nutrients it needs to perform all of its functions smoothly. A typical argument against supplements is that a healthy diet can supply all we need of these nutrients. This may be true of those who live in ideal conditions, with clean air and water, a diet composed only of whole, fresh, organic foods grown in mineral-rich soil, and who don't suffer from much stress. The rest of us must contend with foods that have been grown in depleted soil and that have lost many of their nutrients from sitting on shelves and being cooked or processed. Pollution, toxic chemicals, and unprecedented levels of stress increase our need for certain nutrients. Nutritional supplements give us the support we need to stay healthy in an environment that is anything but healthful.

Research supporting the value of a high-quality multivitamin in the prevention of disease is piling so high that even its most vocal opponents are being forced to admit that it can't hurt and may even help. For example: according to a study recently published in the *Western Journal of Medicine,* about 20 billion hospital health-care dollars a year could be saved if all adults supplemented their diets with folic acid and vitamin E. Folic acid is important for prevention of neural tube defects and premature births, which cost hospitals millions of dollars a year. Vitamin E supplementation is one of the most important steps you can take to prevent heart disease, the number one killer of Americans and the source of huge expenditures for high-tech surgeries and drugs. Extensive research has also been done on the preventive value of supplementing with vitamin C, the B vitamins, the carotenes, the flavonoids, and minerals such as magnesium and calcium.

Here are your basic guidelines for vitamin and mineral supplementation. Try to find a brand that supplies these dosages in two to six pills per day. If you can't swallow pills, powdered varieties are available.

Vitamins

Vitamin A: 1,000–5,000 IU
Beta-carotene or mixed carotenoids: 10,000–5,000 IU

The B vitamins:
  B_1 (thiamin): 25–100 mg
  B_2 (riboflavin): 25–100 mg
  B_3 (niacin): 25–100 mg
  B_5 (pantothenic acid): 25–100 mg
  B_6 (pyridoxine): 50–100 mg
  B_{12} (cobalamin): 100–1,000 mcg
  Biotin: 100–300 mcg
  Choline: 25–100 mg
  Folic acid (folate): 400 mcg
  Inositol: 100-300 mg
Vitamin C: 100–300 mg
Vitamin D: 100–400 IU
Vitamin E: at least 100 IU

Minerals

Boron: 1–5 mg
Calcium (citrate, lactate, or gluconate): 100–500 mg (women should take 600–1,200 mg daily; they can get the additional amount from a calcium-magnesium supplement, discussed below)
Chromium: 200–400 mcg
Copper: 1–5 mg
Magnesium (citrate or gluconate): 100–500 mg (women should take 300–600 mg daily; see below)
Manganese (citrate or chelate): 10 mg
Selenium: 200 mcg
Vanadium sulfate: 25–200 mcg
Zinc: 10–15 mg

Along with your multi, take extra vitamin C (for a total of 1,000–2,000 mg a day), extra vitamin E (for a total of 400–600 IU a day), and a formula of 600 mg calcium and 300 mg magnesium. You can take the calcium-magnesium before bed—it will relax you and help you sleep.

6.
Find a Physician Who Is Open to Alternative Medicine

There is a crisis of faith in Western medicine. Tens of millions of people every year spend more money on alternative health choices than on conventional medicine. Those who seek health want to prevent disease, not just suppress symptoms with drugs and surgery when it's too late to heal.

As people become better informed about how their dietary choices and the use of supplements and preventive medicine affects their overall health, they are likely to find themselves in disagreement with their physicians (and insurance carriers) about the best way to treat an illness. Conventional physicians have been taught that tests, drugs, and surgeries are the best medicine. Most have had barely rudimentary education about nutrition and are focused on diagnosing a disease and giving you a prescription drug to treat it.

Many people complain that their physicians don't treat them as equals, that they are only interested in writing a prescription and getting them out of there to make room for the next patient. This isn't necessarily the physician's fault; he or she is under enormous financial pressures and time constraints. Managed care is reinforcing the "diagnose and medicate" mindset in the medical profession. Many insurance carriers won't cover alternative treatments, and most HMOs won't use physicians who embrace these methods for healing. Enjoying optimal health means going against the grain and perhaps paying out of pocket for alternative health services—at least until insurance carriers add these services to their plans. Some already offer coverage for nutritionally oriented, acupuncture, or chiropractic treatments, but they are few and far between.

To find a physician open to alternative health, including nutrition, in your area, try contacting one of these organizations:

The American College for Advancement in Medicine
P.O. Box 3427
Laguna Hills, CA 92654
(800) 532-3688; in California, call (714) 583-7666

The American Holistic Medical Association
4101 Lake Boone Trail, Suite 201
Raleigh, NC 27607
(919) 787-5146

7.
Find Natural Alternatives to Prescription and Over-the-counter Drugs

A recent article in the *Journal of the American Medical Association* estimated that 140,000 Americans die each year from adverse drug effects, or ADEs. This puts ADEs near the top of the list of leading causes of death in the United States. Another study, this one from the FDA, stated that each year, approximately 938,000 Americans suffer "injuries" as a consequence of prescription drugs. Taxpayers and health insurance holders pay billions of dollars a year for the treatments and hospitalizations that result from these injuries. This doesn't take into account the subtle but significant changes in quality of life caused by side effects of prescription drugs.

In many instances, one drug's side effects are treated with another drug. This is the "drug treadmill." Many people who get on this treadmill end up feeling terrible, but would never think to attribute this to the effects of the drugs they use. Drug-related deaths and injuries are often the result of polypharmacy—the administration of several drugs to the same person at the same time. Mistakes in the dispensation of prescription drugs and drug interactions also contribute to the problem. Where do you think the real war on drugs needs to be waged?

Meanwhile, drug companies are getting richer and taking control of the health care system. They sponsor continuing education for physicians, buy HMOs, and publish biased studies about their latest wonder drugs. One of the most insidious tactics of the drug companies is their attempt to medicalize aging—establishing the notion that menopause is a disease to be treated with estrogen, that aging women should use powerful "designer estrogens" to prevent breast cancer, or that it's a matter of course to put aging people on blood pressure and cholesterol-lowering drugs. The considerable risks of these drugs are downplayed and their potential benefits trumpeted in full-page, glossy advertisements in leading medical journals, magazines, and newspapers. Imagine the earning potential for the drug companies if the entire baby-boomer population were to end up taking multiple medications from their fifties onward.

If you wish to avoid being caught up in this mess, adopt a three-pronged tactic. First, find a physician sympathetic to your wishes to stay off prescription and over-the-counter drugs. Second, if you already take any medications, talk to your physician about weaning yourself off of them as much as possible. When you go to your doctor, be prepared to ask him or her about any alternative treatments you've read about. (If you are using medications, please don't discontinue them without your doctor's help.) Third, if you absolutely must use a prescription drug, be as informed as you can possibly be about what it does in your body, its possible side effects, and any interactions it may have with other drugs or foods. Be sure you are given the lowest effective dose. Watch for errors carefully—know the generic and brand name of your prescription, and check every time you have it filled to be sure you're getting the right drug.

8.
Add Movement to Your Daily Life

For some of you, exercise is a four-letter word. When you think of exercise, you might think of donning tight-fitting workout gear to slog away on a treadmill, or some other activity involving a great deal of sweat and strain. The latest research indicates, however, that mild to moderate exercise is every bit as good for your health as intense exercise. It's actually better for you to take a pleasant walk than it is to suffer through an exercise session that you hate. The most important thing is that it's something you enjoy and that you will do consistently for the rest of your life. Whether that's walking, running, swimming, dancing, bicycling, martial arts, rock climbing, or any other mode of activity is up to you.

This isn't to say that you shouldn't challenge yourself a little in your exercise program. When you go for your walk, for example, you should go at a brisk enough pace to bring out a light sweat and speed up your heartbeat. If you haven't exercised in some time, you may need to begin slowly and build up.

The best and simplest exercise is walking. All you need is a safe route and some walking shoes with plenty of cushioning and support. Covering a half mile is certainly better than sitting on the couch, and walking a mile or two is better yet. Aim for three to four miles, four to five times a week. Give yourself plenty of time to reach this goal; go gradually. Once you're able to log three to four miles in an hour on a flat surface, try a hillier route. Keep challenging yourself, gently, and your fitness level will improve and your exercise will stay interesting.

Three times weekly, use weights, rubber tubing, or your own body weight to strengthen your muscles, connective tissues, and bones. This is called resistance exercise. Stretch to keep joints supple. You can stretch after walking, and whenever else you think of it: as you sit in front of the television, read, or stand in line. Yoga, Tai Chi, and Chi Gong classes are terrific for staying limber and strong. Check into the many books and videotapes available to help you learn proper form for strengthening and stretching exercises. Attending a few classes or hiring a trainer for one or two sessions should be enough to get you started.

You can improve your fitness level simply by adding more movement to your everyday life. Park as far as possible from the store and walk. Ride your bicycle or walk rather than driving when you can. Take the stairs instead of the elevator. Make housework and gardening an opportunity to bend, twist, reach, and squat rather than a chore. The important thing to remember is that your body was made to move, and it works best when you move it regularly.

9.
Pay Attention

Next time you're about to pop a sugary snack into your mouth, stop for a moment. Are you really hungry, or just feeling in need of a little comfort food? Are you acting on force of habit, munching out of boredom? Or is it the time of day you always have a sweet snack? Perhaps you would gain just as much satisfaction from a tall glass of water, a piece of fruit, or a walk around the block. Take the time to listen to your body. If you listen for those subtle messages, your body will tell you what it needs.

The point here is to become aware of what you are doing. This doesn't mean you will decide against gobbling down that candy. You may well decide that despite it being bad for your body, you're going to eat it anyway. Be attentive after you have eaten it, as well, noticing the consequences of having had a concentrated dose of refined sugar.

This works in every area of your life. It isn't about punishing yourself for being "bad"—it's about simply noticing your habitual behaviors and the way those behaviors mold your life. If you remain attentive and aware of what you are doing and why, you'll find it easier to make healthy choices.

10.
Manage Stress with Healthy, Loving Relationships, Community, and Spiritual Practices

An emerging science called psychoneuroimmunology is confirming what holistic, alternative medicine has known from the beginning: your thoughts, feelings, attitudes, and relationships have quite a significant effect on how well your body functions. For example: when we are depressed, upset, or in mourning, our immune systems are severely compromised, making way for disease. This is how people die "of a broken heart." We can decrease our heartbeat and blood pressure if we quiet ourselves and meditate. When a person is told by a doctor that he has only a certain number of months or days to live, that person dies right on schedule if he believes the doctor—and tends to live much longer if he doesn't. The placebo effect is an excellent illustration of the role belief plays in the healing process. How else could we explain the fact that a sugar pill appears to cure a wide variety of illnesses about 30 percent of the time?

To attain and maintain optimal health, we must cultivate healthy, open relationships with family and friends. Human beings need to feel as though they are a needed part of their community. Joining local organizations, volunteering, and other meaningful work can help us to live longer and enjoy a better quality of life. Interpersonal struggle is par for the course in any meaningful relationship, but we must be able to deal with the stress of conflict and work both within ourselves and in cooperation with others to find resolution. The best way to remain balanced in the midst of difficult situations is to make some kind of spiritual practice a regular part of your life.

It doesn't matter whether you choose to attend religious services, meditate, take Tai Chi or Chi Gong lessons, yoga classes, or engage in some other practice that links body, mind, and spirit. The important thing is that you quiet your mind, let go of your worries, and reestablish your center so that you know what is really true, what is right, and what is important. Regular spiritual practice

changes your whole outlook on life and diminishes your
unhealthy physical responses to stress. And if a serious illness does catch up with you, a spiritual practice will give
you the tools to cope with those stresses and to marshal
your body's own healing powers.

What Is Arthritis?

The word *arthritis* means "inflammation of the joints." There are over one hundred types of arthritic disease, some of which affect only the joints and others that have more widespread effects. In this book you'll learn about the two major types of arthritic disease: *osteoarthritis,* also known as *degenerative* arthritis; and *rheumatoid* arthritis, also known as *autoimmune* or *inflammatory* arthritis. Almost all of the arthritic diseases fall into one of these two categories. The onset, progression, and symptoms of rheumatoid arthritis and osteoarthritis are quite different, and they usually affect people in different age groups. Later in this chapter, you'll discover exactly how these kinds of arthritis differ, what characteristics they share, and which arthritic conditions fall into each category.

Here are the stories of George, a sixty-two-year-old retired mechanic, and Angela, a twenty-seven-year-old graduate student.

George's Story

George is a young-looking sixty-two, a self-made man who has worked hard to get to a comfortable retirement. He has a full head of white hair and intelligent brown eyes.

"I was in good health through my fifties. I played a lot of tennis, went running a couple of times a week, and ran my car repair business. The only problem was that I had some pain in my knees and hips after I exercised. I didn't think much of it, figured it was just part of getting creaky with passing years. But it got to the point where I couldn't run at all without terrible pain, and my tennis game was suffering. I knew I had to keep active to keep my heart healthy. So I went to see the doc and told him I needed some help. He ran some tests and turned out I had arthritis pretty bad in both knees and in one hip. He offered me this new arthritis wonder drug and said it was the best choice because it wouldn't irritate my stomach. I was all for that. So I took the stuff, and you know, it just didn't work for me. I was still hurting and my stomach *did* hurt. When I went back the doc said, 'Well, it looks like for now you may just have to scale down your activity, and take Tylenol as you need it for the pain.' That sure as heck wasn't the answer I wanted, but I also didn't want to be dependent on medicine. I don't believe in taking medicine, anyhow.

"I looked into the vitamins and things that are supposed to help and tried a couple of them, and they didn't do much good, either. I felt like I was flushing hard-earned money down the toilet. My doc says that if I don't lay off the running and tennis, I can expect to need knee replacement surgery within the next few years. I don't want that, but I don't want to feel like an invalid either."

George has osteoarthritis, the most common kind of arthritic condition. Osteoarthritis afflicts up to 80 percent of people over the age of fifty and up to 10 percent of people worldwide. Forty million Americans are now suffering from mild to severe joint pain and deformation caused by this disease. Many of them are told that they must either live with the pain and joint degeneration or take drugs with dangerous side effects. Surgery is often the last resort for severely degenerated joints.

Angela's Story

Angela, a pretty, petite young woman with blonde hair and a determined gaze, is deeply committed to her psychology studies. Despite her illness, she plans to continue with school until she has earned her Ph.D. Here's her story:

"In the middle of writing up my master's thesis, I started to feel like I was coming down with something, maybe that flu that was going around. I had a low fever for a few days, and I was so tired and weak I just went straight to bed. I didn't want to eat and my muscles were aching. After the fever went away, the pain and stiffness in my joints—especially in my hands, my wrists, and my feet— seemed to be getting worse. When my boyfriend massaged them for me, he said they felt odd, sort of spongy and soft. I remember my hands were so painful that I had to ask friends to type my paper for me. Getting out of bed in the morning was the worst part. I had to ask my housemate to help me get my clothes on a couple of times, the stiffness was so bad.

"At the student health center they took some blood samples, and soon I got my diagnosis: rheumatoid arthritis, or RA. I'd never heard of it and so I asked a lot of questions. I sat there listening and I just started crying. I felt like I'd been given a lifetime prison sentence. According to the doctors, rheumatoid arthritis could cause me to have severe chronic pain, deformed joints, and could eventually cause me to go blind or to have heart failure. 'Is there any cure?' I asked, and the doctor shook her head, looking at me as though I were a helpless victim. I hated that helpless feeling most of all, that sense of 'Why me?' They said in some people it comes and goes, and in some people it comes only once and never returns, and in some it never goes away. 'There isn't any way to predict the course of the disease, and we don't really know what causes it,' they told me.

"The doctors told me that drug therapy for RA has progressed by leaps and bounds, and that the right drugs could keep the disease in check. They gave me a drug that was supposed to control the pain and inflammation in my joints. It worked, but next thing I knew I had to go back to the doctor because of burning in my stomach. They said that those drugs sometimes can cause ulcers, and they added a drug to decrease the acid in my stomach. My pain was only under control for a few months, though, and they switched me after that to a steroid drug and a drug to suppress my immune system, which they said was attacking my joints and causing all this pain. It was really starting to feel like a bad dream. Since then, I've gained twenty pounds from the steroids, I can't sleep, and I'm just feeling rotten all around. So now it's a catch-22: the drugs are making me sick, too, but if I stop taking them I'll be crippled . . . and there really isn't any guarantee that the drugs will keep me out of a wheelchair in the long run."

Rheumatoid arthritis strikes three to five times more women than men, and it primarily affects young people—those between twenty and fifty. Infants and children can also suffer from RA. A total of about three million Americans have been diagnosed with this disease, which is most common in Westernized countries and all but unknown in less developed nations. Some people with RA recover from their first bout and never have it again. Others have long periods of remission between flare-ups, and some struggle against the disease more or less constantly.

If you are reading this book, it's probably because you or someone you care about has some kind of arthritic disease. Whether you're reading up on osteoarthritis or rheumatoid arthritis, these pages contain information and advice to help you make decisions about its treatment and management. You may find yourself skipping over certain sections to focus on whichever type of arthritis you have, especially in chapters 3, 6, and 7. Throughout the book, you'll be told when information applies to one specific type of arthritis. In other chapters, you'll find that most of the information can be applied to either rheumatoid or osteoarthritis, perhaps with some slight variations.

Arthritis Basics

Now that you know a little bit about the typical course of the two most common kinds of arthritis, let's look deeper into the workings of your joints. Knowing how your joints work, and about what can go wrong with these marvels of engineering, is a prerequisite to knowing how best to support their health. Once you've learned the basics you'll be able to grasp the rest of the information in this book much more easily, and you'll also be able to talk more easily with your doctor about managing your arthritis.

Connective Tissues

Arthritic diseases affect the body's connective tissues. Connective tissues are all made up of *collagen* molecules, which are composed of long strands of protein wound together to create a strong, fibrous rope. Collagen is laid down in various gridwork patterns, providing a framework for other proteins, minerals, and fluids to fill in. When collagen fiber grids are filled in with minerals, it creates bones; when they are filled in with varying amounts of other proteins and fluids, cartilage, tendons, ligaments, fascia, and membranes are the result.

The entire human body is held together by connective tissues. Fasciae hold the muscles and organs in place and in their proper shapes. Ligaments attach bones to one another. Fat, which is actually a kind of connective tissue, cushions and supports the organs and bones. Tendons are dense, strong strips of connective tissue that connect the muscle to the bone, a continuation of the fibrous sheath that wraps around the muscle. Other connective tissues, called *cartilage, synovial membranes,* and *bursae,* also provide cushioning and lubrication between the ends of bones.

Cartilage is dense, firm, and almost plastic in texture. It can withstand a great deal of pressure, and springs right back to its original shape when the pressure is removed. Cartilage is a living, growing tissue. It is made by cells called *chondroblasts,* which make protein and carbohydrate substances (*proteoglycans*) that fill in the spaces in the collagen meshwork.

Synovial membranes line the inside of joints and secrete thick, viscous synovial fluid. In a healthy joint, the inner layer of the joint capsule produces just the right amount of synovial fluid, which keeps the joint surfaces lubricated—much the same role that motor oil has in an engine. Synovial fluid also carries nutrients into cartilage and keeps the cartilage surfaces of the joint separate from one another. The capsule's outer layer is bound tightly to the bone. Some joints, such as the knee and the jaw, include cartilage discs that divide the synovial fluid into two compartments.

Bursae create cushions between the bones and the skin.

Tendon sheaths, a kind of bursa, wrap around tendons and secrete lubricating fluid for easy movement of tendons as muscles contract and release.

The most freely movable joints in the body, including the bones of the fingers and hand, the toes and foot bones, and the shoulder, elbow, wrist, knee, and hip joints, are the most likely to develop osteoarthritis. Because they are the most used, they are most likely to become worn down. Rheumatoid arthritis, which has much less to do with wear and tear, most commonly affects the small joints of the fingers, feet, and toes.

Rheumatoid Arthritis

In rheumatoid arthritis, the immune system loses its ability to distinguish between self and not-self. The immune system's entire purpose revolves around being able to make this distinction, but in the case of this and other autoimmune diseases, it errs too far on the side of caution—destroying healthy tissues because they are perceived as foreign.

Scientists know this because of the way the immune system behaves in joints affected by RA. The very same immune cells that target and kill off cancer cells, bacteria, viruses, and fungus are the ones that eat away at synovial membranes, cartilage, bone, and other connective tissues in RA.

Inflammation and Your Joints

When a part of your body becomes red, swollen, painful, and hot to the touch, it's inflamed. So are injuries such as an infected cut, a sprain, or a bump on the head. If bacteria or viruses infect your airways, you're likely to end up with bronchitis, an inflammation of the bronchial tubes. A fever is a full-body inflammatory response. In every case, inflammation is the body marshalling its healing forces to fix something it perceives to be broken.

Modern medicine is still discovering new aspects of this process. We know that in inflammation, the first thing that happens is some kind of injury. It could be an infection, an injury, or some other harmful substance doing the damage. In response to the injury, specialized hormones send out signals to the immune system. *White blood cells* and other immune cells travel to wherever the injury or infection has occurred, killing off and devouring the remains of bacteria, viruses, or other toxic substances.

Histamine: A chemical called *histamine* is released from immune cells called *mast cells* when tissues are damaged. Histamine signals the body to send more blood and fluid to the injured or infected area, causing swelling. Pain receptors are stimulated by histamine and other chemicals released during the inflammatory process.

In any instance where inflammation strikes, the immune and hormonal systems of your body are working together to increase blood flow and immune activity in the injured area. This is a response designed to accelerate the healing process, but when it escalates out of control it can have the opposite effect. We're learning more about how this happens, especially about the role of the foods we eat in maintaining the balance of pro-inflammatory and anti-inflammatory biochemicals in the body. You'll find out more about this in chapter 4.

Free Radicals: An especially dangerous part of the inflammatory process is the formation of *free radicals.* In chapter 1, you read about the importance of minimizing the oxidation of fats in your body by eating healthy fats and by taking plenty of antioxidant nutrients. Free radicals are formed rapidly when an inflammatory response gets rolling. This means that antioxidant support is especially beneficial for rheumatoid arthritis patients.

Autoimmune Response: Runaway inflammation is found in such autoimmune diseases as inflammatory (rheumatoid) arthritis, Crohn's disease (of the large intestine), and Graves' disease (of the thyroid gland). An autoimmune response is the body mounting an immune attack on its own tissues, creating inflammation that often destroys those tissues in the process. It isn't known for sure what causes autoimmune disease, but as you read further you'll find out about strong evidence pointing to poor diet and environmental toxins. There is also a genetic component; if you have family members with inflammatory arthritis, your chances of developing it are greater.

Where RA Srikes

Chronic inflammation can cause widespread damage. In RA, the immune attack is on the joints, sometimes spreading to other parts of the body. It tends to come and go, with periods of intense pain and inflammation alternating with periods of remission. The disease starts out in the synovium, the lining of the joint capsule that secretes viscous synovial fluid. From there, inflammation spreads to the cartilage, bone, muscles, tendons, and ligaments. Deformity and disability are not uncommon in those with RA.

The hand, finger, and foot joints are most commonly affected, usually in a symmetrical pattern. If the right hand and foot are affected, for example, the left hand and foot probably are, too. Stiffness in the affected joints may go away in an hour after rising in the morning, or may last all day. Those with severe RA may need help with personal hygiene, dressing, eating, and bathing.

Carpal tunnel syndrome, tenosynovitis (inflammation of the sheaths that wrap around the wrist and finger tendons), bursitis, general weakness, and anemia (abnormal blood cell counts) are common in RA sufferers. A general feeling of being unwell, muscle pain, weakness, and low-grade fever are also typical early in the course of the disease.

Affected joints become weak, and they can be injured more easily. Inflammation around the eyes may cause tear ducts to deteriorate, leading to dry, itchy eyes. Small *rheumatoid nodules* are found on the tendons of RA patients, and these nodules can also form in the lungs, the eyes, or on the heart muscle. (These nodules aren't harmful, but their presence allows physicians to diagnose RA more accurately.)

Inflammation of the blood vessels (*vasculitis*), of the sac that surrounds the heart (*pericarditis*), or of the lungs (*pulmonary fibrosis*) can also occur in severe RA, and can be life-threatening.

Types of Autoimmune Arthritis

There are several other diseases that fall into the category of autoimmune arthritis:

Ankylosing spondylitis is caused by autoimmune attack on the joints of the spinal column. It affects about 300,000 Americans, but doesn't usually become severe enough to be completely debilitating. It does cause chronic inflammation, which can lead to painful *sciatica* (irritation of the sciatic nerves that run down the legs) or *spinal stenosis* (where the spinal canal closes in on the nerves of the back, causing pain). Numbness, pain, and weakness in the legs also can occur. The main symptom of ankylosing spondylitis is lower back stiffness and pain, especially in the morning, that persists for more than three months. A genetic link has been found to this type of arthritis, and it often strikes people who have inflammatory bowel disease (IBD).

Lupus, also known as *systemic lupus erythematosus* or SLE, is the diagnosis when connective tissues throughout the body become inflamed. The effects of this rare autoimmune disease vary widely from person to person and can include exhaustion, achiness, nausea, joint and muscle stiffness and aches, extreme sensitivity to sunlight, kidney disease, blood disorders, hair loss, problems with mental function, susceptibility to infection, or inflammation of the heart or lungs. The first noticeable symptoms are a butterfly-shaped rash on the face, neck, and arms, along with fever, weakness, and weight loss. In most cases, the disease goes through periods of flare-ups and remissions, but doesn't go away completely. SLE strikes women nine times more often than it strikes men, usually when they are between the ages of twenty and fifty. People of Asian, African, or North American Indian descent are more likely than Caucasians to develop SLE.

Gout is caused by a disorder of *uric acid* metabolism. Uric acid is a normal product of the body's processes, but in the case of gout, uric acid crystals build up in the body. They become lodged in the joints, and the immune system attacks them. Drinking too much alcohol, being obese, and having high blood pressure increases the risk of gout.

Psoriatic arthritis is associated with the skin disease

psoriasis, which is also thought to be an autoimmune disease. The inflammation that causes the skin irritation spreads to the joints.

Reiter's syndrome is a mysterious disease that affects the eyes, urinary tract, and joints, primarily striking young to middle-aged men.

Sjögren-Larsson syndrome is an autoimmune disease that affects moisture-producing glands throughout the body. Severely dry mouth, eyes, and skin are the most prominent symptoms, and joint pain and inflammation are often involved as well.

Conventional treatments are similar for all of these types of autoimmune arthritis. There is a third category of arthritic diseases—*infectious* arthritis. Infectious arthritis is caused by bacteria, and the symptoms may be similar to autoimmune arthritis. If you visit the doctor with the symptoms of autoimmune arthritis, he or she will rule out the possibility that they are being caused by bacteria. Infectious arthritis is usually treated with antibiotics.

Osteoarthritis

Osteoarthritis (remember that "-itis" means "inflammation of") rarely involves inflammation, and so the name "arthritis" isn't exactly appropriate for this joint disease. Some members of the medical community have begun to use a different term—*osteoarthrosis*—instead.

In most cases of osteoarthritis, the cartilage that has cushioned joints for a lifetime becomes worn down and frayed. Chemical changes result in the loss of two types of connective tissue fibers—collagen and proteoglycans (the protein matrix that fills in the collagen gridwork). In aging cartilage, protein-digesting enzymes dramatically increase their rate of activity, leading to rapid deterioration of cartilage. The body can't replace it fast enough, especially an aging body that doesn't make cartilage as well as it used to.

Men are much more likely than women to develop osteoarthritis young, but women are ten times more likely to develop it than men after the age of forty-five. Nearly every person over the age of sixty-five shows some evidence of cartilage deterioration, especially in the weight-bearing joints of the hips, spine, and knees. Only about a third of them ever have arthritis symptoms, however. This is a good indication that there are factors in play in osteoarthritis that have little to do with the amount of cartilage in the joints. Although we don't know exactly what those factors are, they may explain why certain natural remedies work to relieve the symptoms of the disease.

Symptoms and Causes

In osteoarthritis, there appears to be a genetic factor at play. Those who develop osteoarthritis in their forties or sooner are likely to have other family members who did the same. This could have to do with family members having similar joint structures that are more vulnerable to wear and tear, or to other factors (which will be discussed in detail in chapter 6).

In those who do develop osteoarthritis, the roughened edges of joints rub against one another, causing considerable pain. Joints become stiff, and they may begin to crackle and pop when they are used. Usually, the pain sets in when the joint is used, and relief comes with rest.

The body attempts to repair the damage done, but usually the new bone and cartilage isn't the right shape or in the right place. Bone spurs form, compounding the friction and pain in the joint. As the joint deteriorates, the synovial membrane becomes irritated and overproduces synovial fluid, causing swelling in the joint spaces. Sometimes this swelling is referred to as inflammation, although it rarely involves visible changes in the joint, and may not produce heat or involve the immune system. The irritation caused by friction between joint surfaces simply causes the synovial membrane to make more fluid than the joint can hold. In advanced osteoarthritis, authentic inflammation—heat, swelling, redness, and pain—sets in as the body strives to heal itself.

Athletes who overuse specific joints, or workers who repetitively perform certain motions for years on end, are susceptible to arthritis in the joints they use most. In some people who develop arthritis, joints aren't put together exactly right, and this causes excessive wear and tear on the cartilage. Imagine trying to screw an improperly aligned lid on a jar—when you turn it, the lid and the jar grind against each other rather than the surfaces gliding smoothly over one another. Poor postural habits can have the same effect, throwing joints out of alignment and causing uneven stresses on cartilage and other connective tissues.

When we don't put our joints through their full ranges of motion on a regular basis, they are prone to osteoarthritis. Cartilage doesn't contain blood vessels and receives oxygen and nutrients in the fluid that bathes the joint. Think of it as a sponge that has to be wrung out and let go repeatedly to rinse away dirt and bring in clean water. In this context, that wringing action is the movement of the joint, and that clean water is fluid containing the nutrients this living tissue needs to thrive.

Osteoarthritis most commonly affects the joints of the knees, hips, shoulders, and lower back. These are the workhorse joints of the body. Other types of osteoarthritis include:

Tendinitis: swelling or inflammation of the sheaths around tendons.

Bursitis: swelling or inflammation of the bursa, fluid-filled pads that cushion joints.

Carpal tunnel syndrome: swelling or inflammation of the sheaths around the metacarpal tendons in the hands.

Fibromyalgia: pain in muscles throughout the body, without any inflammation.

Tendinitis and bursitis are often the result of sudden stresses or injuries. Carpal tunnel syndrome is caused by overuse of the joints in the hands, and the cause of fibromyalgia is still somewhat of a mystery.

Now That You Know What Can Go Wrong . . . Let's Look at Solutions

Many people think a diagnosis of arthritis means taking a lot of over-the-counter or prescription drugs, along with inevitable pain and disability. If you have been under this impression, keep reading—there's good news ahead. There is a lot more you can do to relieve arthritis symptoms and slow the progression of joint destruction. The sooner you take action on your own behalf, the less likely your disease is to progress to the point where it becomes disabling.

There has been a lot of hype around so-called "natural cures" for arthritis. Articles and books have boasted that certain supplements can reverse the damage arthritis does to the joints. If you are a conscientious health-care consumer who tries to keep up with the latest research, you may have tried some of these therapies, despite the fact that many are dismissed as useless by conventional medicine. Some may have helped you, and others may have had no effect. Either way, you may feel a bit confused by all the choices available to you.

You'll find out about the choices conventional medicine has to offer—how they work, what risks they carry, and what their track record has been so far. You will also find out all you need to know about alternative medicine's answers for arthritis. Specific nutritional approaches, exercise tips, and tools and techniques for dealing with chronic pain will also be covered in detail. Knowing the facts will help to guide you toward the right regimen for your body and your lifestyle.

The solutions in this book are not miracle cures, although some people do enjoy complete relief when they try new approaches. However, rest assured that if you apply the information in these pages, you will be able to improve your overall health, partly or completely relieve your symptoms, and enjoy enhanced quality of life.

Always keep in mind that improving your overall health is the single most important thing you can do to control arthritis. The conventional medical approach to disease tends to look at the human body as a series of unrelated systems, as though it is a machine with exactly the same components working in the same fashion. According to this approach, disease is the result of one of these systems malfunctioning, and the way to fix the problem is to do a patch job on the system that's breaking down. This book embraces a *holistic* perspective of health and healing. Your body is, indeed, a holistic organism—composed of integrated, interdependent systems, not an assemblage of independently working parts. You can't heal a single part of the body if the rest of it is out of balance.

3

Conventional Medicine and Arthritis

Arthritis is classified as a chronic disease. This means that there isn't any known way to cure it. It may go away without treatment, it may come and go, or it may be a constant part of everyday life, but we haven't figured out how to cure it with drugs or medical technology. It shares the dubious honor, along with heart disease, diabetes, cancer, asthma, and allergies, of being one of the chronic diseases on the rise in Westernized countries. Just when modern medicine conquered most life-threatening infectious diseases in the middle of the twentieth century, the problem of chronic disease began to escalate. It continues to do so at an alarming pace.

Conventional medicine's approach to defeating infectious disease involves finding the offending organism and killing it with a powerful drug, or fending it off with a vaccine. This approach doesn't work with chronic diseases. There is almost never a single, isolated factor that causes chronic disease. Complex factors including diet, lifestyle, genetics, and levels of stress and physical activity all come together to produce fertile ground for a chronic disease to take hold. Reversal of all the processes that went into creating that environment in the body requires a great deal more than a "magic bullet."

I don't intend to completely dismiss conventional medicine's tools for treating arthritis, however. In order for the health-care system to work at its best, allopathic (conventional) and alternative medicine must work collaboratively, with each having a solid understanding of the other's practices. If we continue to operate from the standpoint of "good guys" and "bad guys," each won't reap the benefits of the huge body of knowledge the other branch possesses and the patient gets shortchanged. There is a place and time for conventional measures, and in this chapter you'll learn more about how to recognize when the benefits outweigh the risks.

That having been said, allow me to point out some of the ways in which conventional medicine has made alternative practices out to be the "bad guys." If you read the Arthritis Association's extensive patient literature, you'll find it adheres to conventional medical approaches almost exclusively. It devotes a few passages here and there to "unproven remedies," basically advising readers to steer clear of supplements and natural treatments. Their reasoning is that even if one of these so-called unproven remedies is harmless, it can cause damage to the body simply because it does not stop the destruction of joint tissues. They warn against some supplements because they have potential side effects and emphasize the fact that not as much research has been done on natural remedies as has been done on prescription drugs. They neglect to mention some key points in their dismissal of natural approaches, however.

Of all the drugs used to treat arthritis, not a single one is free of the potential for side effects—and those caused by drugs are far more serious than those caused by natural remedies. This fact is glaringly obvious to anyone who reads the Arthritis Association's literature about the drugs commonly used to treat arthritis. They also don't mention the new "fast-track" approval system for prescription drugs, which allows drugs to go on the market after minimal testing, or the fact that, according to the *New England Journal of Medicine,* prescription drug errors and side effects kill at least 140,000 Americans a year. If any nutritional supplement manufacturer had that kind of track record, you can bet the FDA would close them down pretty quickly.

There is evidence, which you'll read more about in the pages to come, that the conventional treatments used for osteoarthritis could cause the disease to progress more rapidly than it would were it not treated at all. This is, of course, not mentioned in the Arthritis Association's consumer information warnings that supplements could be harmful if they don't actually control or reverse the disease. When you also consider that conventional treatments are not effective for everyone, this particular argument against natural medicine for arthritis loses its clout.

Several studies have sought to trace the natural progression of osteoarthritis. The researchers conducting these studies followed their subjects for years, charting the progression of the disease without giving any kind of treatment. In one of these studies, nearly half of the patients who had advanced hip arthritis recovered without any medical intervention. Their bodies were able to reverse the course of the disease. It is also known that many of the biochemical changes that go on in joints affected by osteoarthritis are geared toward repairing damaged tissues and restoring the function of those joints. This is good evidence that the best we can do for osteoarthritis may be to give the body the raw materials it needs to do this job on its own—with the right diet and supplements—rather than loading it up with drugs.

In the case of rheumatoid arthritis, which can pose the threat of permanent joint deformity, the use of medications and surgery may be necessary to deal with episodes of severe inflammation. You'll find, however, that there are dietary changes, supplements, and natural remedies that can make a difference, even when they are used along with conventional treatments.

Why Natural Is Safer than Synthetic

It's quite rare that anyone suffers any type of side effects from supplements or natural remedies. This is because they are substances that occur in nature that work in harmony with the body's complex systems. Drugs, which are natural molecules altered in laboratories, are designed to potently affect a single variable in one of those systems. The slightest alteration in the structure of a natural molecule can create a substance with a much more powerful effect on human physiology. Increased power of action means increased risk of adverse effects.

Drug manufacturers are usually aiming for the greatest possible *specificity*. When a drug has specificity, it works to alter a single biochemical reaction in the body, without affecting other reactions. The problem with this is twofold. On the one hand, if a single system is affected—if the "magic bullet" hits its mark exactly—it creates an imbalance with other systems that should be integrated with it. This imbalance could cause drug side effects.

It rarely happens that a drug is absolutely specific. What more often causes drug side effects is *lack* of specificity. If the "magic bullet" doesn't exactly strike its mark, it affects not only the system it's aimed at, but other interdependent ones as well. For example: one class of drugs is designed to relieve joint inflammation by inhibiting the production of certain biochemicals. These substances belong to a larger class of biochemicals, some of which are important for other body functions. The drugs aren't specific enough to inhibit only those that cause inflammation. They inhibit the whole class, and adverse effects are the result. This is the case with the most commonly prescribed drugs for arthritis, the nonsteroidal anti-inflammatory drugs (NSAIDs). You'll find out more about these drugs as you read on.

You may have found yourself caught in this crossfire yourself as you have tried to make the best choices for your own health. It might help you to know that the politics and economic issues surrounding pharmaceutical companies, the medical industry, and physician education have considerable influence on what information reaches physicians and the public. Money from pharmaceutical interests funds much of the medical research done in this country. Pharmaceutical companies have little desire to pay for research on nutritional supplements. Natural substances can't be patented, and so drug companies can't name their prices and make huge profits the way they can by altering natural substances and patenting them for use as drugs.

This is not to say that there aren't unethical supplement manufacturers out there who are trying to sell you something worthless. Supplements are big business.

That's why it's so important to find information you can trust, and to be able to talk with your doctor about whether a natural remedy could work for you. There are some wonderful manufacturers of nutritional supplements who maintain rigorous standards of quality based on excellent research. It's simply a matter of separating the wheat from the chaff. The government isn't going to do it for you.

During the last decade of the twentieth century, arthritis drug research and development has become a major emphasis for the pharmaceutical industry. There's an enormous market for anti-arthritis drugs that promises to continue growing with the aging of the baby boomers. Many who are prescribed these drugs are expected to take them for the rest of their lives. That's a lot of money in drug company coffers. This chapter will help you to sort out the hype and the facts about these drugs, so that you can make clear decisions about how your arthritis will be treated.

Conventional Drugs and Therapies

The drugs used to treat arthritic conditions fall into three major categories: *nonsteroidal anti-inflammatory drugs,* or NSAIDs; *corticosteroid drugs;* and *disease-modifying antirheumatic drugs,* or DMARDs. Each type of drug works to relieve inflammation and pain, but each does so by different mechanisms. Let's take a look at each class of drugs, their risks and benefits, what they are prescribed for, what other drugs they can have harmful interactions with, and what their side effects can be. In later chapters, you'll discover how natural substances can do the work many of these drugs do, with gentler action and less risk of side effects.

As you read through this chapter, keep in mind that most drugs have more than one name—a chemical (generic) name and a brand name. Acetaminophen, for example, is sold under the brand names Tylenol, Acephen, Neopap, Redutemp, Arthritis Foundation Pain Reliever, and others. If you buy a generic version, it will simply be labeled as acetaminophen. All of these drugs are the same. Because there are so many brand names for each drug discussed, they will usually be referred to by their generic names. Make sure that you know the chemical name of any drug you are taking; if you aren't sure what that name is, ask your pharmacist.

All You Need to Know about Eicosanoids

Nonsteroidal anti-inflammatory drugs (NSAIDs) relieve arthritis symptoms by inhibiting biochemicals that are thought to play an important role in pain and inflammation. In 1872, the first of the NSAIDs—aspirin—became a popular remedy. Dozens of other NSAIDs have been developed since then. Because NSAIDs pose high risk to the gastrointestinal tract when used for extended periods, physicians have had to be judicious in their use for chronic diseases. In the late 1990s, drug companies developed new NSAID drugs, including celecoxib (Celebrex) and rofecoxib (Vioxx). In order to understand how these drugs work, you'll need some basic information about some of the physiological processes involved in inflammation and pain, and about how NSAID drugs affect them.

All of the NSAIDs work by influencing levels of biochemicals called *eicosanoids* (eye-KAH-suh-noyds). Eicosanoids are a special kind of hormone. Instead of being secreted by glands into the bloodstream, the three types of eicosanoids are secreted by cells throughout the body. They act upon the cell that made them and on other cells in that area. Their effects are incredibly far-reaching, influencing almost every physiological process.

- *Prostaglandins* modify immunity, pain responses, inflammation, body temperature, the constriction and expansion of blood vessels, the clotting of blood, and the health of the lining of the stomach, kidneys, and small intestines.
- *Leukotrienes* (LEW-koh-TRY-eens) modify inflammation and immunity as well as mucous secretion and muscle contraction.
- *Thromboxanes* (thrahm-BOX-aynes) modify blood clotting and pain responses.

There are several types of prostaglandins, several types of leukotrienes, and several types of thromboxanes, and they have balancing effects on one another. For example, there are prostaglandins and leukotrienes that cause inflammation, and others that stifle it. There are thromboxanes that encourage the clotting of blood, and others that thin the blood and prevent clotting. Maintaining the proper balance of each class of eicosanoid is an important aspect of staying healthy. NSAIDs bring down fever and control pain and inflammation by affecting the formation of these locally acting hormones.

Eicosanoids are built out of fats. The "bad" eicosanoids that encourage inflammation and intensify the sensation of pain are mostly built from *arachidonic acid,* the type of fat found in red meat and dairy products. They can also be made from *omega-6 fats,* which are found in most nuts, seeds, and vegetable oils. *Omega-3 fats,* which are found in fish, walnuts, pumpkin seeds, and flaxseeds, are transformed only into "good" anti-inflammatory and pain-relieving eicosanoids. Omega-6s can also be made into the "good" eicosanoids. However, it's important to remember that the labels "good" and "bad" aren't entirely accurate, because inflammation, blood clotting and blood thinning, mucous production, and pain are all a necessary part of the healing mechanisms of the body. What we're looking for is a balance of these hormones, not to totally suppress any of them.

The amounts of these various fats in the diet influence the balance of eicosanoids—you'll learn more about this in the chapter on diet—but this balance also hinges upon the presence of certain enzymes.

There is an enzyme called *cyclooxygenase,* COX for short, that does the actual mechanical work of transforming fats into prostaglandins. Wherever these transformations are going on, two types of COX enzymes are present: COX-1 and COX-2. COX-1 is needed to make the prostaglandins that protect the kidneys and GI tract. COX-2 is needed to make the prostaglandins that increase inflammation and pain. Another enzyme, *5-lipoxygenase,* is needed to make the leukotrienes that increase inflammation.

Older NSAID drugs inhibit the action of both types of COX enzymes, which is why they are dangerous to the GI tract and kidneys. Newer *COX-2 inhibitor drugs* have greater specificity for the COX-2 enzymes, which, in theory, means that they pose far less danger of adverse effects. These drugs have been widely advertised as "super aspirins."

Nonsteroidal Anti-inflammatory Drugs

Aspirin and other NSAIDs are valuable remedies for *occasional* aches, pains, or inflammation. NSAIDs are available over the counter and in stronger versions by prescription.

If you're taking any of these medications, you're taking an NSAID:

> *Aspirin and other salicylates, including:*
> choline salicylate
> diflusinal

magnesium salicylate
salicylsalicylic acid
sodium salicylate
sodium thiosalicylate

Ibuprofen and similar drugs, including:
diclofenac
etodolac
fenoprofen
flurbiprofen
indomethacin
ketoprofen
ketorolac
meclofenamate sodium
mefenamic acid
nabumetone
naproxen
oxaprozin
piroxicam
sulindac
tolmetin sodium

COX-2 inhibitors, including:
celecoxib (Celebrex)
rofecoxib (Vioxx)

Some pain relievers combine a salicylate or acetaminophen (see below for more on acetaminophen) with
sleep-inducing drugs, muscle relaxants, caffeine, or diuretics. Drugs sold under the brand names Midol, Ex-
cedrin, Pamprin, Anacin, Cope, Extra Strength Tylenol
Headache Plus, Fiorinal, Esgic, Butace, Amaphen, and
Lanorinal are examples. Any drug that contains NSAIDs

should state the generic name of that NSAID clearly on the label.

In the early stages of arthritic disease, conventional medicine treats a stiff, painful joint caused by autoimmune attack in much the same fashion as a stiff, painful joint caused by injury or overuse. Since RA is an inflammatory disease, it makes sense to treat it with anti-inflammatory drugs. These medications are often effective at relieving the pain of osteoarthritis, despite the fact that it rarely involves inflammation. The question is, do the benefits of NSAIDs outweigh their risks?

NSAID Side Effects

When these drugs are used on a daily basis, as they often are in arthritis, risk of adverse effects rises dramatically. Ulcers and gastrointestinal bleeding caused by NSAIDs kill at least 10,000 people *every year* and are the reason behind at least 76,000 hospitalizations yearly. (I'll explain how these drugs cause ulcers in a later section of this chapter.) The ulcers caused by NSAIDs are especially dangerous because the painkilling action of the drug masks the discomfort they cause. Pain is the body's only way to warn us of early development of an ulcer. Once bleeding becomes noticeable—it can appear in the stools or can appear in the form of vomit that looks like coffee grounds—the ulcer is a serious threat. As with many prescription drugs, these drugs are also dangerous to the kidneys.

Even if NSAIDs don't cause such serious problems, they can cause a more subtle condition called *leaky gut*. The shortage of "good" eicosanoids (particularly some types of prostaglandins) causes tiny holes to erode in the intestinal wall, allowing partly digested food and toxins into the bloodstream. As soon as these substances get through the intestinal wall, the immune system tags them as foreign and attacks them. If this constant stress on the immune system goes on for very long, the immune system gets confused about what to attack and when to stop.

Leaky gut sets the stage for chronic diseases such as severe allergies, asthma, and autoimmune diseases like rheumatoid arthritis. The symptoms of these diseases are caused by an overactive immune system, one that has lost the ability to turn itself off when it should. It isn't recognized by conventional medicine, so don't be surprised if your doctor has never heard of it. If you see a naturopathic doctor or other type of complementary medical professional for treatment of allergies, asthma, or rheumatoid arthritis, he or she will likely suspect leaky gut.

NSAIDs are only one possible cause of leaky gut. It can also be caused by food allergies, which will be covered in more detail in chapter 4. Also, look to that chapter for an explanation of how the use of acid-reducing medications for NSAID-caused ulcers can work against the body's efforts to heal damaged joints.

If you are using salicylates, also look out for side effects such as nausea, upset stomach, stomach pain, heartburn, or blood in your stools. Such side effects can mean that you're developing an ulcer or gastrointestinal bleeding and should be attended to by a physician right away. Other side effects to look out for with salicylates include rashes, hives, anemia, easy bruising and prolonged bleeding (due to their blood-thinning effects), and ringing in the ears (tinnitus). They have also been associated with detachment of the retina and macular degeneration, the leading cause of blindness in the United States.

Be very wary of using salicylates if you have kidney disease, and always stop taking aspirin or other salicylates a few days before any kind of surgery to avoid excessive bleeding. Taking an aspirin an hour before having an alcoholic drink raises blood alcohol levels 26 percent higher than they would go without the aspirin. If you are using anticoagulant drugs (blood thinners), carbonic-anhydrase inhibitor drugs for glaucoma, methotrexate (prescribed for rheumatoid arthritis and other autoimmune diseases), loop diuretics, or ACE inhibitors, be aware that taking aspirin or other salicylates with these drugs can cause potentially dangerous drug interactions.

If you are using ibuprofen or similar drugs frequently, be aware that nausea, vomiting, heartburn, diarrhea, constipation, gas, cramps, or bloody stools could be the result of their use. Urinary tract problems, including increased infections and frequent urination, hepatitis, and jaundice can be side effects of these drugs. Other possible side effects include dizziness, drowsiness, headache, fatigue, nervousness, depression, vision, weight or blood pressure changes, mineral imbalances, menstrual problems, male impotence or breast enlargement, and anemia. Stay away from these drugs if you are scheduled for surgery, or if you have kidney or liver disease, any history of GI inflammatory disease (such as inflammatory bowel disease or Crohn's disease) or ulcer, anemia, pancreatitis, eye disease, infection, or extreme sensitivity to sunlight. Ibuprofen and similar drugs can have health-threatening interactions with anticoagulant drugs, lithium, methotrexate, ACE inhibitors, beta blockers, loop diuretics, thiazide diuretics, and DMSO (a nutritional supplement, sometimes used to treat arthritis; see page 127). Always take NSAIDs with food to minimize stomach irritation.

Another downside of NSAIDs is their effect on a hormone called melatonin. Melatonin is made in a tiny gland in the brain called the pineal gland. When night falls, melatonin is secreted to send out the message that it's time to sleep. Children, teenagers, and young adults make plenty of melatonin and their sleep quality is usually very good. As we age, melatonin secretion drops, and we have more trouble going to sleep and staying asleep. This can be compounded by NSAID use. In one study, a single dose of aspirin decreased melatonin production by up to 75 percent.

COX-2 Inhibitors: Hope or Hype?

As is the case with any new drug that sounds too good to be true, there is more to know about the "super aspirins" than the drug companies may want you to know.

There has been an amazing amount of hype surrounding these drugs. Arthritis sufferers have gone to their doctors in droves to ask for them, thinking they will be more effective than the NSAIDs they've been taking. The truth is that the COX-2 inhibitors have not been proven more effective against arthritis pain than the older NSAIDs. There's no evidence that Celebrex or Vioxx will relieve symptoms the other NSAIDs aren't able to relieve.

Although they do appear to pose less danger of side effects, it's clear that more research is needed before this is known for certain. The COX enzymes have so many functions that it's impossible to know the ramifications of inhibiting one of them until the drug has been thoroughly tested (which it hasn't been). We know that COX-2 plays an important role in the body's ability to repair damaged tissues and in maintaining proper blood flow through the kidneys. The result of suppressing this enzyme long-term remains to be seen. Another consideration: the COX-2 inhibitors are also extremely expensive—around three dollars a dose.

NSAIDs Slow Cartilage Healing

Even if the new NSAIDs were completely harmless to the GI tract, there is another very good reason for osteoarthritis patients to try to steer clear of NSAIDs in general for long-term use: these drugs interfere with the body's ability to repair cartilage. Dozens of studies published in leading medical journals have shown this to be true. Some leading researchers have good evidence that these drugs actually accelerate the progression of osteoarthritis.

It's hard to understand why a responsible health-care professional would prescribe anti-inflammatory drugs for a joint disease that rarely involves inflammation except in its advanced stages—especially when they carry such substantial risks and slow the healing of cartilage. They do relieve pain, but there are plenty of other ways to achieve this end.

Rheumatoid arthritis is a different story. Because it's primarily an inflammatory disease, NSAIDs might be a necessary evil—at least temporarily—to prevent joint damage. Not treating out-of-control inflammation is a high-risk proposition. There are natural remedies and nutritional changes that will decrease inflammation, however, and you'll find out about those in chapters 6 and 7.

Acetaminophen

Acetaminophen is a painkiller and fever reducer. Best known as Tylenol, it reduces pain by affecting the transmission of pain messages through the nervous system. It's used most in osteoarthritis patients who have difficulty with NSAIDs.

Some who have stomach troubles from NSAIDs or are allergic to aspirin are led to believe that acetaminophen is a safe alternative. It isn't as safe as it's made out to be, because of the considerable danger it poses to the liver. Drinking alcohol, using other drugs in combination with acetaminophen, or even just using it a little bit more often than recommended can permanently damage the liver.

Even the recommended doses can put considerable stress on liver function. In chapter 4, you'll discover how important the health of your liver is to the health of your joints (and to the rest of you).

Other possible adverse effects with acetaminophen include fever, hypoglycemic coma, low white blood cell count, easy bruising, and excessive bleeding. Acetaminophen can also interact dangerously with lithium, ACE inhibitors, beta blockers, and loop diuretics. If taken with barbiturates, carbamazepine, hydantoins, rifampin, or sulfinpyrazone, the risk of severe liver damage increases dramatically.

NSAIDs and acetaminophen are known as "first-line" treatment for osteoarthritis and rheumatoid arthritis. What happens when these drugs fail to control symptoms adequately? Conventional medicine brings out the big pharmaceutical guns: corticosteroids and disease-modifying antirheumatic drugs (DMARDs). Corticosteroids given by mouth and DMARDs are reserved for the treatment of inflammatory types of arthritis. In osteoarthritis, corticosteroids injected directly into painful joints are the last resort short of surgery.

Corticosteroid Drugs

Cortisol is a steroid hormone made in the adrenal glands. Steroid hormones, a class that also includes progesterone, DHEA, testosterone, androstenedione, and the estrogens, are made from a hormone called pregnenolone, which is made from cholesterol. Without cortisol, the body cannot cope with stress. Technically speaking, we can survive without cortisol in the body, but the moment any kind of stressor enters the picture—hunger, fear, illness, or any kind of strenuous physical activity—we would become very sick or die without sufficient output of cortisol.

Now, let's say you're constantly under stress, taking in too much caffeine, and overexercising. All of these circumstances lead to increased cortisol production. This hormone's effects are widespread: heart rate and breathing speed up, blood flow is diverted away from the digestive tract and to the muscles, and stored sugars are mobilized and passed into the bloodstream, quickly raising blood sugar levels. The activity of the immune system is suppressed. In other words: too much cortisol isn't a good thing, either.

Synthetic Cortisol: In 1949, drug researchers developed synthetic versions of cortisol, such as prednisone. They are similar to natural cortisols, but are not found in nature, and thus can be patented. Synthetic cortisol drugs are also much more potent than those made in the body, and small doses have pronounced effects and equally pronounced side effects. The natural cortisols were replaced with the synthetic ones for economic reasons (drug companies can charge more for patent drugs) and were prescribed to treat the symptoms of inflammatory diseases and allergies. It has become common practice to call all the cortisol-related hormones made by the adrenals, as well as the synthetic versions, "cortisones," but this is inaccurate. Cortisone is a specific hormone that must be converted in the body to cortisol before it is active. In this book we'll refer to cortisol and related hormones, including the synthetics, as corticosteroids.

A common treatment for rheumatoid arthritis is oral (taken by mouth) synthetic cortisol, such as prednisone. For osteoarthritis, it is injected into affected joints to provide relief from pain and swelling. When injected into the joints, cortisone can stave off pain for up to a few months, but because the injections are very damaging to cartilage and bone, they can't be given frequently.

Corticosteroid Side Effects: Soon after the synthetic oral corticosteroids prednisone and prednisolone went into widespread use, it became obvious that they were not without serious side effects. When used for more than two weeks, synthetic cortisone drugs can cause significant weight gain, sleeplessness, water retention, mood swings, personality changes, high blood pressure, increased risk of infections, yeast infection, cataracts, glaucoma, acne, growth of facial hair in women, osteoporosis, aseptic bone necrosis (where parts of bone tissue don't get adequate blood flow and die—a very serious problem that can destroy joints permanently), diabetes, and inflammation of the pancreas (pancreatitis). Steroid drugs are a major cause of osteoporosis in women—just a few injections over a period of a year can cause steep drops in bone mineral density.

Synthetic corticosteroids should always be used in the smallest possible doses for as short a period of time as possible. Only natural cortisol (usually sold as either hydrocortisone, cortisol, or Cortef) should be used long term. For anyone taking corticosteroid drugs for any length of time, the book *Safe Uses of Cortisol* by William McK. Jefferies, M.D., should be required reading. It details how using natural cortisol in physiologic doses (those that mimic what the body would make) can be very safe and effective for a wide range of problems, including a variety of types of arthritis.

Another problem with long-term synthetic oral steroid use is dependency. If synthetic cortisones are put into the body day after day, the adrenal glands get lazy and stop making cortisone. If the drugs are stopped abruptly, symptoms of withdrawal and even death can result. Those who have had to use these drugs long term must taper their doses gradually. They are strongly encouraged to wear a medic-alert bracelet or pendant in case of an accident, because any physician who works on them will have to take special precautions. The least stress can severely injure someone who doesn't make enough cortisone. Increased vulnerability under stress lasts for up to two years after discontinuing the medication. Synthetic corticosteroid drugs can have dangerous interactions with salicylates (aspirin), isoniazid, antacids, barbiturates, phenytoin, and rifampin.

If you must use synthetic corticosteroid drugs, try to do so for less than two weeks at a time. Encourage your doctor to give you the smallest possible dose. In some patients, it can be used every other day rather than every day.

Usually, low-dose corticosteroids for RA are tried if NSAIDs don't work. The next course of action is the disease-modifying antirheumatic drugs (DMARDs). If the DMARDs don't stop the disease from progressing, patients are put on higher doses of corticosteroids.

Disease-Modifying Antirheumatic Drugs

These drugs are reserved for the treatment of rheumatoid arthritis that can't be controlled with NSAIDs or low-dose oral steroid drugs. If you are taking any of the following drugs, you're taking a DMARD:

methotrexate
hydroxychloroquine
chloroquine
gold (auranofin)
sulfasalazine
azathioprine
etanercept (Enbrel)
leflunomide (Arava)

The DMARDs are also known as *slow-acting rheumatic drugs,* because they can take anywhere from one month to one year to become effective. Methotrexate works the most quickly, usually in a month to six weeks; auranofin can take from six months to a year to become effective. Most of the other drugs in this class take from three to six months to kick in. They may be given orally or by injection. As medical researchers search for a cure for RA, they uncover new immune factors that seem to have significant actions in the disease. Once those immune factors are identified, pharmaceutical companies race to develop drugs to target them.

Traditionally, DMARDs have been reserved for use only when other measures fail to control inflammation in RA, but the most recent trend is to use them earlier to prevent permanent damage. They can be effective at stopping the progression of the disease and preventing joint damage, but as soon as the DMARDs are stopped, the symptoms return. Their often severe side effects prevent 30 percent of patients who take them from continuing long enough to gain the benefits in the first place.

It isn't known exactly how some of the DMARDs work. Many are believed to jam up the cellular equipment that drives the inflammatory process. Some of the DMARDs work by shutting down certain immune system functions, interrupting the cascade of events that leads to uncontrolled inflammation.

DMARD Side Effects: Here are some of the side effects that may occur with the use of these medications:

Methotrexate: Ulcers and bleeding in the mouth and throat; vomiting; intestinal cramping; bloody or non-bloody diarrhea; painful urination; bloody urine; reduced resistance to infection; severe depression of immune cell formation in the bone marrow; kidney, liver, and lung damage; loss of hair

Hydroxychloroquine: Light-headedness; blue-black skin, mouth, or fingernail discoloration (with long-term use); nausea; vomiting; stomach cramps; diarrhea; hair loss or loss of hair color; headache; visual blurring; serious damage to corneas and retinas of eyes; severe depression of immune cell formation in the bone marrow; heart muscle damage; ringing in ears or hearing loss.

Auranofin (oral or injected gold): Diarrhea; liver damage; jaundice; skin rash; sores in mouth and on tongue; nausea; vomiting; stomach cramps; headache; partial or complete loss of hair; cough; shortness of breath; drug-induced pneumonia or lung damage; blood cell and bone marrow toxicity, leading to fatigue, sore throat, and abnormal bleeding or bruising; pain, numbness, and weakness in arms and legs (*peripheral neuritis*); side effects from this drug can surface months after the drug is discontinued.

Azathioprine: Increased risk of infection; increased risk of cancer; suppression of immune cell formation in bone marrow; rash; vomiting; diarrhea; sores in mouth and on lips; liver damage; jaundice; drug-induced pneumonia.

Two newer drugs have been introduced for the treatment of RA that don't respond to the other DMARDs. Leflunomide (Arava) is a newer DMARD that has a mode of action and side effects similar to those of methotrexate—but without the lung toxicity associated with the latter drug. Etanercept (Enbrel) is one of the newest DMARDs, having been approved in 1998. It works by inhibiting the binding of *tumor necrosis factor* (TNF) to receptors. When TNF binds to receptor sites, it triggers the formation of pro-inflammatory prostaglandins and other inflammatory cells. Blocking this reaction decreases joint inflammation in between 60 and 75 percent of those who use it.

The most common side effect of Enbrel is swelling and irritation at the injection site, which in early studies occurred in 37 percent of patients. It dramatically increases the risk of infection—35 percent of patients in the clinical trials developed upper respiratory and sinus infections. More serious infections, including bronchitis, infectious arthritis, wound infections, pneumonia, and sepsis (a deadly infection in the bloodstream), become more likely with the use of this drug. It stifles the action of an anticancer arm of the immune system, which may lead to increased risk of cancer. Its cost is quite high, earning the drug companies $10,000 per year per patient. Both Arava and Enbrel are often given in combination with methotrexate.

All of these medications are dangerous on their own, but can become even more so when taken with other drugs. Anyone using them must work in close communication with his or her rheumatologist and should not put any drug—over-the-counter, recreational, or prescription—into his or her body that hasn't been checked out with the physician first.

A decision to use any of the DMARDs is a difficult one. Their side effects can be devastating, and they don't work for every RA patient. In those patients who do respond to these drugs, relief from their disease might make the side effects worthwhile. But it's important to give natural approaches a try before resorting to such powerful medications, as soon as the disease is diagnosed. With the right diet and supplements, RA sufferers can often either postpone or avoid the need for these drugs.

Antibiotics for Arthritis

Since the 1930s, some arthritis experts have tried to prove that most cases of rheumatoid arthritis are caused by bacteria. Successful cures have been achieved in small studies where antibiotics were given to rheumatoid arthritis patients. The research in this area is definitely intriguing, but hasn't been consistently supportive of this theory.

Antibiotic therapy for rheumatoid arthritis is still in its experimental stages. It isn't likely that your doctor will recommend it to you until a lot more research has been done. This theory has resurfaced and been disproven so many times and the risks that accompany chronic antibiotic use are so serious that the likelihood of antibiotics becoming conventional therapy for rheumatoid arthritis is small.

Surgery for Arthritis

When a joint ravaged by osteoarthritis or rheumatoid arthritis loses its mobility or causes uncontrollable pain, surgery is often recommended. The type of surgery you have will depend on which joint is to be repaired and what kind of damage has been done to that joint.

Arthroscopy: In this type of surgery, the surgeon uses a very thin tube—an arthroscope—with a tiny light and camera at its tip. It's inserted through a small incision near the joint and allows the surgeon to have a look around to see how much damage has been done. A tool can be threaded through the arthroscope to cut away loose cartilage or to smooth down roughened joint surfaces. Recovery is quick and usually no hospital stay is needed.

Osteotomy: In osteoarthritis, bone can grow irregularly or can become misshapen. Osteotomy is the surgical removal of deformed bone to improve the function of a joint.

Resection: Removal of part or all of one of the small bones in the foot, wrist, elbow, or thumb when osteoarthritis causes severe deformity or pain.

Arthrodesis: When joints are beyond repair, the two

halves can be fused together. The joint is no longer movable but becomes much less painful and more stable. Usually this surgery is done on the joints of the thumb, ankles, wrists, or fingers. In some instances of arthritis in the backbone, vertebrae are fused together.

Arthroplasty: Also known as joint replacement, arthroplasty is a last resort for arthritic hips, knees, shoulders, elbows, ankles, and knuckles. The surgeons replace the degenerated joint with an artificial one. This type of surgery is serious and entails at least a week's hospital stay and outpatient physical therapy, but in many cases can rescue patients with advanced arthritis from becoming invalids. It's a good thing these procedures exist and are relatively safe and effective, but all possible measures should be taken to prevent the disease from progressing this far. The older and feebler the patient is, the greater the risks involved with arthroplasty.

Synovectomy: This surgery involves the removal of diseased synovial tissues from joints of RA patients. The synovium does grow back, and the procedure often needs to be repeated within a few years' time. This procedure is done with an arthroscope.

The decision to have surgery is a major one. Be sure you have a second opinion before agreeing to it, and if at all possible have outpatient surgery to avoid a hospital stay. Hospitals are not safe places for sick people. They are crawling with antibiotic-resistant infections, and misprescribed drugs kill tens of thousands of hospital patients every year. Going under general anesthesia is a risky proposition. Being in the hospital and the fear of going under the knife can be stressful all by themselves, not to mention the actual stress your body goes through while you're having the operation and starting your recovery.

If you do have to go to the hospital for your surgery, be

sure to prepare yourself adequately. Here are some guidelines for you to follow if you will be having inpatient surgery. You should advise your doctor of any supplement, vitamin, or drug you are taking prior to surgery.

- Support your liver, which will have to process a great many drugs during your surgery and your recovery. The herb milk thistle (use as directed on the container), alpha lipoic acid (200 mg three times a day with meals), and N-acetyl-cysteine (500 mg three times a day with meals) all promote the health of the liver. Use these nutrients for one week prior to and two weeks after surgery. (If you are diabetic, be aware that alpha lipoic acid can cause blood sugar levels to drop; start out with 50 mg twice a day and build slowly, and let your physician know you are using it.) Also, get plenty of fiber in your diet to keep your bowels moving—constipation interferes with good liver function.
- Improve your immune system function before going into the hospital. Vitamin A (not its precursor, beta-carotene) is the best choice for improving immune function. Take 15,000 IU a day for the week before surgery, 50,000 IU a day for the two days before, and 15,000 IU for about ten days following. If you are pregnant, don't take more than 15,000 IU a day. Also, take 1,000–2,000 mg of vitamin C, 200 mcg of selenium, and 15 mg of zinc—*in addition* to your regular daily supplements.
- If you are taking salicylates or other NSAIDs, which thin the blood, discontinue them at least a week before surgery. You should be able to continue taking 400 IU a day of vitamin E, which is a mild blood thinner. Check with your doctor to make sure.

Follow this plan for the two weeks before and two weeks after surgery.

Bioflavonoid antioxidants, such as green tea extract or grapeseed extract, are useful after surgery to speed healing. Follow the instructions on the container. The amino acid glutamine helps your body de-stress and detoxify, and aids in good digestion. Use 500 mg twice a day, for a total of 1,000 mg, between meals, for a week before and two weeks after your surgery.

Learn relaxation techniques to help you cope with stress and pain before, during, and after your hospital stay. See chapter 8 for some helpful tips.

The Arthritis-Busting Diet

In chapter 1, you read about a basic plan for a truly healthy approach to eating, which is to focus on whole, fresh foods and avoid processed foods. This is not an approach that rides the wave of any fad, but one that is natural, common sense, and uncomplicated. It isn't a miracle weight loss diet to help you melt off the pounds or erase wrinkles, although you may well find yourself trimmer and younger-looking once you've followed the guidelines for a while. It isn't even about curing any disease, although you may find that nagging chronic joint pain will decrease or disappear and that you get sick a lot less in general.

Eating primarily whole foods is not an extreme diet—although it may seem so at first if you're accustomed to the Standard American Diet (SAD), where ketchup and french fries are considered vegetables and where most food and drink has been stripped of nutrients and is full of added sugar, salt, flavorings such as MSG, and preservatives. This dietary advice is designed to give you variety, to teach you to appreciate the tastes and textures of whole foods, and to give you enough leeway to occasionally enjoy sweets.

In this chapter, you'll learn more about how food can be good medicine for both osteoarthritis and rheumatoid arthritis. Furthermore, eating in a way that supports joint health provides the right environment in your body for any arthritis treatment plan to be as effective as possible—whether you decide to use conventional medical approaches, natural approaches, or a combination of the two.

Many people have asked some version of this question: "Why should I think that my diet has anything to do with my arthritis, when I've eaten this way all my life and didn't have arthritis until now?" A youthful body can usually handle a diet of processed foods, because its digestive and cleansing mechanisms are in peak condition. They can efficiently process what you eat and flush out toxins. As you age, those mechanisms don't function as well and need a little more care and attention. A suboptimal diet also has cumulative effects over a lifetime, so that the adverse effects may not show up until your fifties or sixties.

The arthritis-busting diet takes a two-pronged approach. First, you'll find out how to restore your body's natural balance with foods that support your digestive and cleansing organs. You'll learn how to safely cleanse your body of toxins that contribute to the progression of joint disease, simply by emphasizing certain foods and avoiding others. You'll also find out about some superfoods that are especially good for people with arthritis.

Biochemical Individuality: No One Diet Works for Everyone

A toxin is any substance that can do damage to living tissue. Some toxins, called *exotoxins* (*exo*=exterior), come into the body from outside. Examples of exotoxins are prescription drugs, chemicals found in the environment, or artificial food additives or preservatives. Even some of the foods we think of as health-promoting, such as milk, tomatoes, soybeans, or wheat, contain natural toxins that some people react to unfavorably.

Other types of toxins, called *endotoxins*, are formed within the body in the natural course of its day-to-day functions. Inflammation and other immune system activities produce toxins that can kill healthy cells. Potentially toxic substances are manufactured by unfriendly bacteria or yeasts that live in the body. A healthy body can easily handle these types of toxins in small amounts.

Toxicity isn't so much about the substance itself, but about the way it interacts with a person's body. Something that is quite toxic to one person can be harmless to another. For example, in a person with a peanut allergy, the most minute bit of peanut protein can kill. The rest of us can eat a peanut butter and jelly sandwich without a second thought. Even poisonous chemicals such as pesticides and herbicides are less toxic to some people than they are to others.

Most of us have a relative who's been smoking and drinking since his teens and who is still going strong into his eighties. Another example of this concept—which science refers to as *biochemical individuality*—is the fact that while one person may suffer debilitating side effects from a drug, another person can take it for years without any problem.

Certain people have bad reactions to toxins when they accumulate beyond what the body can process. Some people can handle more than others. A complex interplay of genetics and one's past and present habits create these differences. The capacity of the digestive organs and the organs that neutralize toxins varies from person to person. During a person's lifespan, subtle changes in the body, diet, or environment can cause new sensitivities to crop up; along the same lines, reactivity to toxins can fade with time.

Diets for Osteoarthritis and Rheumatoid Arthritis: How Do They Differ?

In osteoarthritis, the right diet supports the repair of damaged cartilage. Taking steps to support the function of your digestive and cleansing organs will help you to get the full value of foods and supplements that support joint health. It's also important for those with osteoarthritis to find a diet that will help drop excess pounds. Obesity is a major contributing factor in this form of arthritis, because it increases stress on the joints.

A diet to slow the progression of rheumatoid arthritis is designed to keep inflammation in check. The concepts of toxicity and biochemical individuality are especially significant in autoimmune arthritic diseases such as rheumatoid arthritis and lupus. Some people are more susceptible to these disorders than others. It could be genetics, stress, hormone imbalances, overexposure to endo- or exotoxins or a combination that triggers an overblown immune response.

The dietary approaches to osteoarthritis and rheumatoid arthritis overlap in many respects. Doing all you can to support your digestive tract and liver is the foundation for any arthritis-busting diet. Here are the essentials on how these organs work, what can go wrong there, and about how your joint health depends upon their proper functioning.

What You Need to Know about Digestion

Your digestive system creates an interface between your body and the environment. The role of this group of organs—also known as the gastrointestinal (GI) tract—is to break down what you eat and drink into its most basic molecular components and to pick and choose what passes through its walls into the bloodstream.

Whatever isn't absorbed has to be disposed of, and this is another part of the job done by the digestive and cleansing organs. Any exotoxins that do get absorbed, along with the endotoxins created inside the body, are—ideally—filtered out of body fluids and disposed of by the liver and kidneys. In ancient healing practices, such as Chinese and Indian (Ayurvedic) medicine, supporting the function of the kidneys and liver is part of healing many illnesses. These organs are among our best allies in the fight against disease, and a healthy, toxin-free diet is the best way to keep your kidneys and liver in good working order. One of the shortcomings of modern drug-based medicine is that damage to the kidneys and liver are common side effects of even the safest drugs.

Let's take a whirlwind tour through your digestive tract, so that you have a good basic understanding of how everything works. This will help you to understand what can go wrong and how the arthritis-busting diet can fix these problems.

The Stomach

The stomach's job is to break down food as completely as possible, so that when it goes into the small intestines, it's ready to be absorbed into the bloodstream and distributed throughout the body. It does so by secreting *hydrochloric acid* (HCl) and a protein-digesting enzyme called *pepsin,* and mixing them into the food with strong contractions. Another ring of muscle separates the stomach from the small intestine. When the acidity of the stomach contents—now called *chyme*—reaches a certain level, that muscle gets the signal to relax. The chyme is then passed in small squirts into the small intestines.

The Small Intestines

Near the mouth of the small intestine lies the pancreas. This small organ secretes enzymes into the chyme to further digest proteins, carbohydrates, and fats. These enzymes dismantle large food molecules, reducing them to their most basic elements, the *macronutrients.* It is these elements—fatty acids (from fats), sugars (from carbohydrates), and amino acids (from proteins)—that are finally absorbed into the bloodstream and distributed to where they are needed. Vitamins, minerals, and other micronutrients are also liberated and absorbed during this part of digestion.

The small intestine is a complex organ, an excellent example of multi-tasking—it's a digestive organ and an immune system organ rolled into one. Its twists and turns are lined with what looks like a microscopic shag carpet. Tiny nubs called *villi* cover its surface, increasing the surface area through which nutrients can be absorbed. Each villus contains a network of capillaries. Capillaries are blood vessels with walls that are a single cell thick, through which nutrients pass to be carried away to wherever they are needed. The small intestines are also lined with a vast array of immune cells, designed to distinguish between what should and should not be absorbed. These immune cells bar entry to whatever they perceive to be potentially toxic.

The Liver

The liver is the largest solid organ in the body, weighing in at about five pounds. Think of the liver as the body's internal sewage treatment plant, filtering wastes and toxins out of the bloodstream and disposing of them. Drugs, alcohol, toxic chemicals, hormones, allergens, used immune cells, and infectious microbes are all processed by the liver. Aside from its detoxification function, the liver also functions in the production of bile (which is needed for the digestion of fats in the small intestines), cholesterol, and blood-clotting factors. It provides storage space for carbohydrates, vitamins, and iron, and converts many vitamins into their active, biologically useful forms.

Let's say you're rushed for dinner one night and have a fast-food hamburger, soda, and fries. The drugs given to the cattle, the preservatives in the roll, the caffeine in the soda, and the pesticide residues on the french fries are absorbed into the bloodstream from the intestines. From there, they are transported directly to the liver through the portal vein. When the digestive tract is working well, and the toxic load isn't too great, the liver can neutralize and dispose of these toxins. If you eat fast food every day, however, the liver can become overworked. The drugs and pesticides may end up sitting permanently in your fat cells, and the caffeine and preservatives may sit in the bloodstream longer. An overburdened liver is especially common among those who frequently use over-the-counter and prescription drugs, alcohol, and caffeine. If this happens, toxicity builds up and contributes to chronic disease. As we age, the liver's cleansing powers decrease. This is one reason why older people are at higher risk for adverse effects from drugs: the liver doesn't clear substances from the bloodstream as quickly, so the drug stays in the system longer.

Glutathione: As the liver neutralizes toxins twenty-four hours a day, seven days a week, it creates loads of free radicals in the process. An important antioxidant, called *glutathione,* is made in the liver to protect it from free radical damage. A shortage of glutathione can spell trouble for the liver, especially when toxic load is high. The Standard American Diet falls far short of supplying adequate raw materials to make glutathione. Glutathione can't be absorbed through the GI tract, and so it doesn't help to supplement the diet with this antioxidant.

Supporting the health of the liver means cutting way back on over-the-counter drugs and alcohol, and eating a whole foods, organic diet. Given the opportunity, the liver can do an amazing repair job on itself—even after years of abuse. Supplements that support the liver include alpha lipoic acid (50 to 100 mg twice a day) and the herb milk thistle (follow the directions on the container). Foods rich in sulfur, such as eggs, garlic, asparagus, and onions, boost glutathione levels in the liver, helping to protect it as it does its important work. For additional sulfur, always a good idea for an overworked liver, you can use MSM (methylsulfonylmethane) or glucosamine sulfate (which has the added bonus of repairing cartilage).

The Large Intestine

As wastes pass into the large intestine (usually referred to as the colon) from the small intestine, the body tries to conserve water and minerals by reabsorbing them through the colon walls. More water and minerals are reabsorbed when you're dehydrated and depleted of minerals. This means that stools get hard and difficult to pass—more reasons for you to drink plenty of water and take a complete mineral supplement.

Our large intestines actually house an entire ecosystem, including *probiotics* (friendly bacteria), yeasts, and less friendly *putrefactive* bacteria. We have a symbiotic relationship with probiotics, which means that we help them and they help us. They have a place to live and plenty to eat—they dine on undigested bits of food and fiber—and they do some valuable work for us in return. Probiotics manufacture B vitamins and vitamin K, which are absorbed into the body through the colon walls. They produce natural antibiotic substances that keep putrefactive bacteria such as e. coli, salmonella, and clostridium at bay, and help to get rid of chemical toxins. Probiotics also make a substance that prevents the growth of cancer cells in the colon.

Whenever something goes wrong in your digestive tract, it's a sign that things are out of balance. Rather than opting for a quick fix with symptom-suppressing medication, which is the usual response to heartburn, ulcers, and constipation, look to the root of the problem and use natural remedies and diet changes to get relief.

The Real Reason
for Heartburn and Ulcers

The acid-producing cells located in the stomach wall produce less hydrochloric acid as we age. Low stomach acid secretion is also found, although less commonly, in younger people. If you tend to feel full or bloated for a long time after meals, or if you tend to suffer from heartburn, you probably are low on stomach acid. Other symptoms that point to low stomach acid secretion are intestinal gas, bad breath, and a coated tongue. Low acid secretion has been found in people with osteoarthritis, chronic muscle cramps, acne, osteoporosis, asthma, autoimmune disease, eczema, and rosacea. This may come as a surprise if you've been under the impression that heartburn is caused by too much stomach acid.

Insufficient stomach acid production means that food has to sit for a longer time in the stomach before it's ready to go on to the small intestines. Sometimes, if food sits for too long, the stomach pushes it back up into the esophagus, mixed with strong acid. Since the esophagus doesn't have a protective mucous lining like the stomach does, it burns, causing an uncomfortable condition commonly known as heartburn. This problem is often made worse by suppressing or buffering stomach acid with antacids or H2-blocker drugs such as Tagamet or Pepcid.

Ulcers, too, were once thought to be the result of excess stomach acid. Now, we know that 90 percent of them are caused by a bacteria called *h. pylori,* which erodes the protective mucous lining of the stomach. This bacteria can also cause heartburn. When testing shows that *h. pylori* is the cause of an ulcer, it must be treated with a combination of antibiotics and bismuth preparations such as Pepto-Bismol. Many other cases of ulcer are caused by chronic NSAID use, and the only way to cure those ulcers is to discontinue the NSAIDs.

The pain of heartburn and ulcers is your body's way of letting you know that something's awry and needs attention. Using medications to block ulcer symptoms may allow the condition to worsen to the point where it becomes life-threatening. Antacids block the absorption of calcium and may cause diarrhea or constipation. Frequent use leads to rebound acidity, where the stomach tries to regain balance by secreting a surge of acid—which often causes the antacid user to reach for another antacid tablet.

Acid-blocking drugs cause mineral imbalances and diminish the absorption of vitamin B_{12}. Indigestion, diarrhea, and constipation are among the more common side effects of acid-blocking drugs. Some acid-blocking drugs impair liver function. Tagamet (cimetidine) may actually aggravate arthritis symptoms.

If the stomach contents aren't acidic enough, protein-digesting enzymes aren't activated there, and this prevents the proper digestion of food and the absorption of nutrients down the line. Creating an unnaturally alkaline (the opposite of acidic) environment in the body stresses the kidneys and has been linked to increased incidence of urinary tract infection. Fortunately, there are natural alternatives you can try for heartburn and ulcers, without risk.

Natural Remedies for Heartburn and Ulcers

If you have an ulcer or suffer from chronic indigestion or heartburn, and you haven't been using NSAIDs, be sure that you're tested for *h. pylori.* Antibiotics are a necessary evil if this bacteria has taken up residence in your stomach. In any case of ulcer, stop drinking coffee and alcohol, avoid tobacco, and find an alternative to NSAIDs.

For heartburn, avoidance of fatty, greasy foods, processed meats, chocolate, alcohol, and sugar should be your first approach. Overeating at meal after meal saps the strength of acid-producing cells. It takes an enormous effort on the part of the digestive tract to process a big meal. Eating only as much as you need is bound to improve digestion. Be aware that extreme stress, obesity, and pregnancy are also possible culprits. Antidepressants, corticosteroids, blood pressure and cholesterol-lowering drugs, NSAIDs, aspirin, estrogens and progestins used for postmenopausal hormone replacement, and ulcer drugs can all cause heartburn. Even clothing that fits too tightly around the waist can be a contributing factor, so it may be time to hand down those pants you wore when you were thirty.

As long as you don't have an ulcer or active heartburn, you can try some of the following approaches to increase your stomach acid secretion. Don't drink hot or cold liquids with meals, because this slows digestion by decreasing output of stomach acid. Instead, have a glass of water (not cold, just room temperature) half an hour before you sit down to a meal. This actually stimulates your stomach to secrete acid. Adding a tablespoon of apple cider vinegar or bitters, such as goldenseal or gentian, to the water will have a greater stimulant effect. Drinks such as Angostura bitters and Campari encourage stomach acid secretion, and a glass of wine likely has a similar effect.

If none of these approaches work to relieve heartburn, go to your health food store for some betaine hydrochloride (betaine HCl). Take it with meals (not while you're having active heartburn), starting out with the lowest recommended dose on the container and working up slowly until your digestion improves. Don't use betaine HCl or apple cider vinegar if you have an ulcer, or if you are using NSAIDs regularly.

Whether your ulcer is caused by NSAIDs or bacteria, licorice extract is a safe and effective herbal remedy that will speed healing and protect your stomach lining from further damage. It does so by increasing the secretion of mucus in the stomach. Be sure to use *deglycyrrizinated* licorice, or DGL, because other licorice extracts can have strong stimulant effects similar to caffeine. Take 300 mg four to six times a day. Other herbal remedies for ulcers include slippery elm and marshmallow root (200 mg four to six times a day of either). Unripe bananas and the juice of raw cabbage also aid in ulcer repair.

Is Your Gut Leaky? Here's How You Can Find Out

In chapter 3, you read about how NSAIDs can create tiny holes in the wall of the small intestines. These holes allow toxins and incompletely digested bits of food to pass into the bloodstream. These are substances that probably would never get through the tightly knit, highly selective boundary of an intact intestinal wall. Once toxins and undigested food particles get into the circulation, immune cells tag them as foreign and attack them. From that point the body may consider perfectly harmless foods as enemies to be attacked.

If toxins become lodged in joint tissues, they could conceivably start an autoimmune response in that joint. This is one theory about how rheumatoid arthritis gets started. A more generalized immune response throughout the body can mean increased sensitivity to toxins in general. It's thought that this could be a contributing factor in severe environmental allergies and asthma.

Food Allergies: Food allergy can cause leaky gut as well. When the body becomes sensitized to a particular food, the intestinal immune system begins to react to it strongly. The inflammation that results can eat small holes into the intestinal wall. Wheat, gluten, yeast, dairy products, eggs, soy, beef, peanuts, and nightshade vegetables (tomatoes, potatoes, red and green peppers, eggplant, tobacco, coffee, and corn) are common food allergens.

You may have noticed that the foods most likely to cause allergies are those that many people eat every day, or even at every meal. Ironically, it's usually the foods you love the most and feel you couldn't live without that you become allergic to. Most food allergens happen also to be found in a great many processed foods. The allergic reaction creates a mild stimulant effect, and so we may feel addicted to these foods.

There is another kind of food allergy, the *immediate* kind that causes sneezing, hives, runny nose, wheezing, watery, itchy eyes, or *anaphylaxis* (a swelling of the airways that can be life-threatening if not treated immediately). Immediate food allergies, usually to strawberries, peanuts, beans, seafood, or dairy, generally occur in children and are often outgrown. Delayed allergies, on the other hand, affect adults and cause more subtle symptoms. It's difficult to connect them to the offending food, because the symptoms may take some time to develop. For this reason, they are referred to as *delayed* food allergies.

Fatigue, hay fever or other environmental allergies (to animal hair or mildew, for example), indigestion, dry skin, dull hair, rashes, and other health problems that can't be attributed to anything else are often the result of delayed food allergy. Although it may not cause you to feel desperately ill, food allergy means never quite feeling your best, and certainly can compromise your quality of life.

The Elimination Diet

Most conventional medical doctors aren't yet aware of leaky gut and delayed food allergies or how to treat them. However, there is plentiful evidence that when people with chronic illnesses take steps to identify food allergens and eliminate them, they experience significant improvements in their health. Fortunately, identifying your food allergies is something you can do on your own with what's known as an *elimination diet*.

Identifying and eliminating food allergens with an elimination diet takes discipline and attention to detail, and a willingness to deprive yourself of the pleasure of eating the foods you love, at least temporarily. It isn't nearly as easy as taking pills to suppress symptoms. Going on the elimination diet will, however, benefit your health immeasurably, will teach you to appreciate new foods, and will guide you to lifelong dietary changes that will encourage your joints to heal. If you have rheumatoid arthritis, the elimination diet is an especially important step for you to take. You'll also find out more about fasting, another effective natural approach to healing rheumatoid arthritis, in a later section.

Start out by continuing to eat your normal diet. Write down everything you eat or drink for a period of ten days. If you eat a lot of processed foods, try to keep good records of the ingredients they contain. For example: if you have a packaged cinnamon roll for breakfast every day, it probably contains wheat flour, milk, and eggs—all common food allergens.

After a week's time, sit down with your diet record and make a few categories: one for foods you eat at every meal; one for foods you eat every day; and one for foods you eat five or more times a week. Now you know which foods you ought to eliminate. Start out by eliminating the foods in all three categories. If you're eliminating wheat, cut out all gluten-containing grains: wheat, millet, barley, spelt, amaranth, kamut, and oats. Wheat is one of the hardest things to eliminate, since it's hidden in so many products, such as soups and even condiments. Rice, corn, and potatoes do not contain gluten.

You may find it difficult to figure out what to eat during the weeks of the elimination diet. Focus on fresh, in-season, organic vegetables and fruit, all the varieties of brown rice (a grain that is usually the staple of a non-allergenic diet), deep-water fish such as salmon, cod, and mackerel, and small servings of free-range chicken. Meat is also okay, although some people are sensitive to beef. Carefully read the labels of any processed foods you choose. Go to your health food store and have a clerk help you stock up on quick, convenient staples such as rice noodles and organic soups. There are many more choices than ever before for people on restricted diets.

A sample day's meals for someone eliminating wheat and other gluten-containing grains and dairy might go something like this:

Breakfast: two poached eggs, fresh fruit salad, and corn grits

Snack: rice crackers or a small handful of raw nuts and seeds

Lunch: organic vegetable soup with toasted corn tortillas and avocado

Snack: raw celery, carrots, and cucumber with tahini (sesame seed paste) dressing

Dinner: baked salmon, brown rice, and a generous helping of steamed greens (chard, spinach, and kale are good choices), with a green salad; have fruit if you crave something sweet for dessert, or enjoy a cup of caffeine-free herbal tea sweetened with honey.

Eat slowly and deliberately. Take small bites, chew your food completely, and enjoy its tastes and textures. Don't fall into the pattern of eating the same foods day after day; rotate your new staple foods and keep experimenting. Of course, you should drink plenty of water throughout the day. Keep a written record of what you eat. Also write down how you are feeling and whether you notice any changes in your symptoms.

After two weeks, it's time for the food *challenges,* where you reintroduce the foods you have eliminated, one at a time. Don't challenge more than one food in a twenty-four-hour period.

Have only the food you're testing at a single meal. If you are trying to discern whether you have an allergy to wheat, have a bowl of plain cream of wheat cereal or cooked wheat berries. If it's dairy you suspect, have a glass of organic milk, and so on. Once your system has had a chance to empty itself of all of the allergenic food, your reaction to it will be more pronounced. Some of the more common symptoms people experience when reintroducing foods on an elimination diet are fatigue, headache, uneven or unusually fast heartbeat, muscle or joint aches, stomach cramps, bloating, diarrhea, gas, constipation, chills, sweats, and rashes. If you have these or other unusual symptoms when you reintroduce a food, there's a good chance you're allergic to it.

You may find that your health improves dramatically once you cut processed foods with artificial flavorings and colorings out of your diet. If this is what you find, and none of the food challenges yields any results, you may have sensitivities not to the foods themselves but to additives, preservatives, and dyes. Many people are allergic to the yellow and red dyes. Avoiding these chemicals permanently is the best solution.

Once you've figured out what foods set you off, avoid them completely for two months. Chances are, you'll feel much better than you did before going on the limited diet. After two months, test the foods again. If you have a

reaction again, go off the foods for six months before trying again. This will allow your body to lose its sensitivity,
and eventually you should be able to enjoy the foods you
eliminated once in a while—but not every day.

If your food allergies have caused leaky gut, there are
some supplements you can use to help your intestines
heal. Glutamine, an amino acid, is the intestinal wall's favorite fuel; taking 500 mg three times a day between meals
will give the gut cells the energy they need to reestablish
a healthy lining. Supplements to control inflammation in
the intestines are also a good idea during an elimination
diet. You'll find out more about anti-inflammatory supplements and natural remedies in chapters 7 and 8, and in
a later section of this chapter you'll learn which foods have
anti-inflammatory effects. Vitamin B_5 (pantothenic acid)
is needed by the intestinal wall to build healthy cells.
Take 500 mg twice a day during the first two weeks of
your elimination diet.

A Note about Nightshade

One popular theory about diet and arthritis involves allergy to the *nightshade* vegetables. This family of vegetables includes tomatoes, potatoes, red and green peppers,
tobacco, and cayenne pepper. Eliminating these foods has
helped people with both types of arthritis. It's thought
that the *solanum alkaloids* in these foods can cause osteoarthritic or inflammatory changes in the joints of
people who are sensitive to them. If you eat any of these
foods frequently, make sure to include the entire family on
your list of foods to eliminate.

Do You Need Supplemental Digestive Enzymes?

If you tend to have gas and lower abdominal bloating after you eat, try using supplemental digestive enzymes. Gas is formed when undigested food is fermented by bacteria in the colon. If you don't make enough stomach acid and digestive enzymes, a lot of digestion remains to be done in the colon—which means a lot of uncomfortable and potentially embarrassing gas will form. In the case of lactose intolerance, the carbohydrates in milk aren't digested at all, and when they hit the colon they cause gas, bloating, and diarrhea.

Intestinal gas is another problem that will probably disappear when you fix your diet. An optimal diet contains plenty of raw foods, which are naturally rich in enzymes. As we digest raw foods, the enzymes they contain help the digestive process along. The heating of foods kills off the enzymes. It follows that if we don't eat raw foods at every meal, we could probably use some supplemental enzymes. (Pasteurized dairy products and juices don't count as raw foods; they've been heated to high temperatures to kill bacteria, and the enzymes are killed off as well.) Going onto a whole-foods diet suddenly will give some people cramps, bloating, and gas. It's important to introduce new foods such as whole grains into your diet gradually, so your body can get used to digesting them.

Fresh papaya and pineapple are both rich in protein-digesting enzymes. You can buy these enzymes in supplement form to take after meals. A full-spectrum enzyme supplement, containing amylase (for fat digestion), lipase (for carbohydrate digestion), protease (for protein digestion), and lactase (for lactose digestion), will give you better digestive support. Pineapple enzyme, or *bromelain,* also happens to be a potent anti-inflammatory. You'll find out more about this use for bromelain in chapter 6.

Yeast Overgrowth

Yeast (*Candida albicans*) grows in the small and large intestines. It normally coexists peacefully with the other organisms there. If probiotic bacteria populations drop, yeast can become overgrown. *Candidiasis* damages the delicate lining of the intestines, contributing to leaky gut and allowing bacteria to pass into the circulation. Yeasts pump out toxic byproducts that can seep through the intestinal walls, and the immune system is forced to constantly work overtime to get rid of toxins released by the yeast.

Chronic, low-grade candida overgrowth is another disorder that has been almost completely overlooked by conventional medicine. Yet, it's well-established that yeast overgrowth is often found in people with arthritis, autoimmune diseases, constipation, irritable bowel syndrome, heartburn, gas, menstrual problems, out-of-control allergies, food allergies, sugar cravings, sinusitis, rashes, fingernail or toenail fungus, and inflammation of the urinary tract. If you have health problems like these that you can't find any explanation for, you may have yeast overgrowth.

What kills off probiotic bacteria and allows yeast to run rampant? One major culprit is the SAD. A diet high in refined carbohydrates (yeast's favorite food) and low in fiber encourages yeast overgrowth and stifles the growth of probiotics. Antibiotics also kill off good bacteria, allowing yeast to flourish, and birth control pills set up hormonal imbalances that allow yeast to flourish. Oral steroid drugs also have this effect. If you have used any of these drugs for any length of time, there's a greater probability of your having yeast overgrowth.

Just as many people dramatically improve their health with elimination diets, many others do so by taking steps to get yeast overgrowth under control. (In fact, many of those who have leaky gut also have yeast overgrowth.) Doing so can only help; it involves changing your diet and taking a few natural supplements. Relief of pain and inflammation in rheumatoid arthritis and osteoarthritis are among the benefits of restoring order to the intestinal ecosystem.

The approach here is simple: cut way down on refined grains and sugar; use a probiotic supplement with *fructooligosaccharides,* the carbohydrate molecules that are good nutrition for friendly bacteria; and wean yourself off antibiotics, birth control pills, and oral steroid drugs. You can find a good refrigerated probiotic supplement in your health food store. Take it according to the directions on the container. Also eat foods fortified with *lactobacillus* and *bifidus* bacteria, such as live-culture yogurt, kefir, unpasteurized miso, and sauerkraut. Bananas are an excellent source of fructooligosaccharides.

Constipation and Joint Health

If you don't have at least one bowel movement a day, you should take steps to relieve constipation. When your bowels don't move regularly, toxins meant to be eliminated quickly sit too long in the colon and can be reabsorbed. Other bowel toxins, when allowed to sit too long, are transformed into carcinogens by naturally occurring chemicals in the large intestine. Constipation can also lead to hemorrhoids (varicose veins in the anus, which can be extremely painful) and diverticulosis (the forming of pouches in the intestines where food can get trapped and cause dangerous infections). Both are the result of straining to evacuate the bowels.

Food allergies, leaky gut, and yeast overgrowth all contribute to the problem of constipation. (These three problems are interrelated and often exist in the same people.)
If you switch to a whole-foods diet, drink your six to eight
glasses of water a day, and treat food allergies and yeast
overgrowth, it's likely that your constipation will disappear. If it doesn't, you can try a fiber supplement. Psyllium husk is a cheap and effective source of fiber available
at your local health food store. Mix one to three teaspoons
of psyllium in a six- to eight-ounce glass of water or juice
and drink it immediately. Follow it with another glass of
water. If you tend to have problems with intestinal gas,
start with a teaspoon or less and build up slowly.

The Anti-Arthritis Diet, Also an Anti-Inflammatory Diet

Although not all arthritis involves uncontrolled inflammation in the joints, a diet designed to help prevent inflammation from setting in promotes health in many
other ways. Inflammation is being linked to a wide variety
of conditions besides autoimmune disorders—from heart
disease to Alzheimer's disease to cancer. We don't know if
it causes disease or if it's an effect of disease, but either way
it makes sense to eat a diet that will help keep potentially
harmful inflammation from spinning out of control.

Pro-inflammatory and anti-inflammatory eicosanoids
(locally produced hormones; if you need a review on this
topic, refer back to chapter 3) are made out of the fats we
consume. If there is an imbalance between certain types of
fat in the diet, there tends to be an imbalance between
pro- and anti-inflammatory eicosanoids. One of the fats
most overconsumed in the Standard American Diet—
those found in meats and dairy products—are the raw

material from which some of the pro-inflammatory eicosanoids are made. Fats from fish, seeds, nuts, and vegetables (yes, vegetables do contain tiny amounts of fat) are needed to make the anti-inflammatory eicosanoids. However, the most important fats to cut out completely are the hydrogenated oils or trans-fatty acids, found in virtually all processed foods, margarines, and vegetable shortenings.

At the same time, it's equally important not to become fat-phobic and try to cut out all saturated fats. You need saturated fats, too—just not in the amounts most Americans eat them. You also need unsaturated fats, but it's important to be sure they aren't rancid.

Cutting way down on sugar and refined grains (white flour, pasta, white rice) is an important aspect of an anti-inflammatory diet. Processed food diets, especially those high in refined grains and sugar, are directly linked to the insulin and blood sugar imbalances that lead to adult-onset diabetes. Adult-onset diabetics have high blood sugar and high insulin levels, both of which are devastating to the body. It's estimated that 6 percent of people over the age of forty-five are diagnosed with adult-onset diabetes, that another 6 percent have it but don't know it, and that another 6 percent are *prediabetic*—they have high blood sugar and insulin levels, but not high enough to be diagnosed with diabetes. One of the ways in which high insulin levels cause damage is by dramatically increasing the production of pro-inflammatory eicosanoids.

Fasting for Rheumatoid Arthritis

Fasting can have remarkable curative effects on rheumatoid arthritis. Abstaining from food and drink (except for water) may seem like a drastic approach to controlling inflammation, but it works. The elimination diet outlined so far also will work to curb the progression of an RA flare-up, but total fasting will yield more dramatic results more quickly.

Any fast lasting more than three days should be supervised by a physician. This is especially true of those who are using medications. Drugs commonly used for rheumatoid arthritis, including NSAIDs and corticosteroid drugs, are likely to cause serious kidney damage if taken during a fast. If you are using medications, you will need to work with a physician to wean yourself off of the drugs you're using before you can fast safely. Some people cannot fast safely at all and are better off simply shifting to a whole-foods, organic diet. During the course of a fast, the physician will monitor your blood pressure and blood levels of *electrolytes* (minerals). If either of these tests show dangerous changes, your doctor will help you terminate the fast properly.

Fasting has been a part of religious observances throughout history and has been used to treat disease almost as long. Ancient Greek medical texts, upon which modern medicine is based in many ways, prescribe fasting for the treatment of a variety of diseases. Not eating for three to seven days may sound impossible and risky, but most humans can go without food for up to forty days without any significant ill effects.

When you undergo a fast, your body has a rare opportunity to reestablish balance, without the stress of digesting and assimilating food three or more times a day. In his book, *Fasting—and Eating—for Health,* Joel Fuhrman, M.D., says it succinctly: "Therapeutic fasting . . . works because the body has within it the capacity to heal once the obstacles to healing are removed."

After the second or third day of a fast, feelings of hunger dissipate, and a shift takes place—the body's energy needs are filled by stored fuel. Internal changes are made to preserve muscle tissue and provide energy from stored fat. This mode is also a cleansing mode. Detoxification processes, relieved of the constant work of processing meal after meal throughout the day, have a chance to clear out stored wastes from body tissues. Liver function and immune system function are both improved during a fast.

Side Effects of Fasting

It isn't uncommon for people who are fasting to experience nausea, headaches, strange body odors, itching, rashes, fatigue, congestion, aches and pains, dark urine, foul-smelling bowel movements, and other unpleasant symptoms. As the body burns up stores of fat, toxins are set loose in the circulation before they are detoxified or excreted, and they can't be eliminated fast enough. They can rise to high enough levels in the body that you'll feel worse before you feel better. The more symptoms you experience, the more toxicity you've been carrying around in your body, and knowing that you're getting it out of your system may be some small consolation. Judicious use of enemas is helpful in the cleansing process, as are dry-brushing the skin before showering and alternating hot and cool water in the shower. While fasting, get as much rest as you can, avoid stress, and take plenty of naps.

It's very important to properly prepare for and break a fast. Two weeks on a whole-foods diet, tapering down to only vegetables, fruit, and rice, is the best way to ease into a fast with the least trauma to the body. At the end of a long fast, you'll need to break it carefully, starting out with small meals of easy-to-digest vegetables and fruits, and cooked whole grains, and adding fats, seeds, and protein foods in gradually, increasing amounts two to three days after the fast has ended.

If a long fast seems too daunting or is impossible for you

because of medications or other factors, there are less drastic approaches you can take. Periodic one-day water fasts are safe for nearly everyone, with the exception of insulin-dependent diabetics. Those who don't wish to go without food can try a one-day to one-week cleansing diet consisting only of fresh organic vegetables, fruit, water, and tea. While extended fasts are more potent medicine than these other approaches, you'll still gain considerable benefit. Another plus for those who wish to try the shorter fasts or cleansing diets: you won't need a doctor's supervision.

An excellent resource on fasting and elimination diets is the book *Optimal Wellness* by Ralph Golan, M.D.

Eat Less, Enjoy Life More

Research is revealing that eating too much food for years on end not only can make us overweight, but can also cause us to age prematurely. Studies of animals and humans with low caloric intakes show that they are far less likely to fall prey to heart disease, cancer, and other chronic diseases. They live longer and have more energy. The research also shows that caloric intake over a whole lifetime is the important thing. Whether we periodically overindulge and make up for it with a fast or simply refrain from overeating in general, we can still enjoy the benefits of longer life and less chronic disease. Eating less also reduces excess weight, which relieves stress on arthritic joints.

5

Exercise
for Pain-Free Joints

Regular exercise is one of the most important steps you can take to slow the progression of arthritis. You may not be able to run marathons, climb mountains, or swim the English Channel, but you can do a lot to keep your joints from losing their range of motion. When joints hurt, the instinctive response is to try to avoid moving them. Unless they're severely inflamed (hot, red, and swollen), you should try to move them to whatever extent you can tolerate.

Maintenance of muscle strength and cardiovascular fitness, relief of pain and stiffness, and better sleep quality are some other good reasons to establish an exercise routine. Whether your arthritis is severe or mild, there is always something you can do to keep moving. By the time you finish this chapter, you'll have all the information you need to design a safe, effective exercise program for yourself.

Use It . . . Don't Lose It!

Your body is exquisitely engineered to move. When we sit for years on end at desks, in cars, or in easy chairs, it begins to protest. If we don't take advantage of the many ways in which we can bend, squat, stretch, lift, and twist, we eventually discover that we can no longer do these things the way we used to. The perils of a sedentary lifestyle are well-known. If you don't get any exercise, your risk of having a heart attack, stroke, and cancer go up, and your chances of being overweight are much greater. Whether you're in your twenties or your eighties, it isn't too late to start exercising now. Even people in their nineties make remarkable gains in strength, flexibility, and overall health once they start an exercise program.

Moderate exercise is especially important if you want to avoid or slow the progression of osteoarthritis. Remember: cartilage doesn't have its own blood flow and is nourished by the fluid that is pumped through it when a joint moves. Without this pumping of joint fluids, cartilage doesn't get the nutrients it needs and can't get rid of wastes and toxins. Excessive exercise that causes repeated strain in the ankles, knees, and hips can cause osteoarthritis, so it's important to take a moderate approach. For those with rheumatoid arthritis, regular exercise is essential for maintaining joint mobility and strength, but care must be taken to avoid overdoing it or injuring weakened or inflamed joints. "Use it or lose it" is appropriate for an arthritis exercise program; "no pain, no gain" is not.

An exercise program for arthritis should include three elements: flexibility, strength, and cardiovascular fitness. First, let's talk about another element that links all three of the others: breathing.

Remember to Breathe

I know this sounds a little bit ridiculous. How could a person forget to breathe, especially when they are exercising and need more air? Check in with your own breathing for a moment. Don't change anything, just watch. When you inhale and exhale, can you see your chest rising and falling? How about your abdomen? Place your hands on your rib cage. How much does it expand and contract with your breath?

Now, try taking a couple of deep breaths. Do your shoulders automatically hike up to your ears? Does it feel relaxing, or does it make you feel tense and light-headed to breathe deeply? Try one more thing. Go to a wall and push against it with both hands. Did you hold your breath while you were pushing?

By now, you probably have a better understanding of what it means to remember to breathe. When we don't pay attention to our breathing, it gets shallow, and the depth of our inhalations and the force of our exhalations become less. The muscles we use for breathing—the diaphragm, a large muscle below the lungs that causes them to expand, pulling air in; the intercostal muscles and the obliques, which expand the ribs wide; and even the muscles across the chest and upper back—become tense and lose their suppleness when we don't practice breathing deeply.

Being aware of the breath and learning to control it is powerfully health-promoting. When we can consciously breathe more deeply and slowly, we can relax the body through pain and stress. Holding the breath or breathing shallowly sends an alarm response through the body, causing it to make biochemicals that create tension. Taking deep, relaxed breaths soothes those responses. Deep breathing is an essential element of ancient forms of exercise such as yoga, Chi Gung, and Tai Chi. Meditation, the process of quieting the mind and body by focusing on the breath, can unleash the body's healing powers in ways that are just beginning to be recognized by conventional medicine.

It's especially important to focus on the breath during exercise. When you strain through an exercise that hurts or is difficult, it's natural to want to hold your breath. This can cause a temporary but marked rise in blood pressure, which can be dangerous for those who have hypertension. Concentrating on breathing slowly and steadily through strength and flexibility exercises will help to make it a pleasure rather than an unpleasant chore.

A Meditation Breathing Exercise

Here is a meditation exercise that will help you to focus on your breathing. Sit comfortably, with your back straight. If it's hard for you to sit straight, sit on the floor on a cushion and lean against the wall, or sit in a straight-backed chair. Imagine that each of the vertebrae in your spine is stacked right on top of the one below it, and that your shoulders and arms are hanging limply from your spine. Don't slouch the shoulders forward or pinch them back. Place your hands palms up on your thighs. Tuck your chin slightly down toward your collarbones, lengthening the back of your neck. Let your sternum (the bony center of your chest) rise slightly toward your chin. Allow the space between your shoulder blades to widen. Sit quietly for a minute or two.

Now, start to focus on your inhalations and exhalations. If your nasal passages are clear, you should do both through the nose. The inhalation should start at the very base of your abdomen, causing it to expand. It then moves up to expand the lower back, the rib cage, and the sternum and upper back. Visualize it as a warm blanket of sunlight climbing up your body and draping over your shoulders. Don't let your shoulders hike up, and don't force your breath deeper than it wants to go. When you have inhaled completely, hold the breath in for two seconds.

Exhale slowly by relaxing all the muscles you used to bring the breath in. Don't force here, either; the exhale should take the same amount of time as the inhale. Exhale as much air as you can and hold the breath there for two seconds before inhaling again. If the holding feels too uncomfortable, you can just take continuous inhalations and exhalations. If you have asthma or emphysema, diseases that can make it difficult to exhale all the air in the lungs, purse your lips through the exhalation and blow the breath out through the mouth, as though you're trying to put out a candle.

Once you get the hang of this, try doing it with your eyes closed, counting your breaths backward. On the first inhale, count fifty; on the first exhale, count forty-nine; on the next inhale, count forty-eight; and so on. When you reach twenty, start only counting the inhalations. By the time you get to zero, you'll feel wonderfully relaxed, alert, and invigorated.

While meditating, allow your mind to be empty. Whenever internal chatter starts going on in your head, let it happen, but always return your attention to your breath. Don't let that internal chatter distract or frustrate you—simply let it go. If you are experiencing pain during your meditation, rather than dodging away from the sensations or tensing up, fully acknowledge the places that are painful. Send your own version of healing energy into them: perhaps a caressing, massaging hand, warm rays of light, or warm water.

Try to do this meditation once each day, at whatever time you need most to relax. Some like to meditate right after rising in the morning, while others use it as a mid-day break. Still others meditate in the evening to unwind from the day.

Cardiovascular Fitness

The accepted facts about cardiovascular exercise—the kind that keeps your heart, lungs, and blood vessels strong—are changing. We now know that it isn't necessary to sweat buckets on the treadmill or jump around in an aerobics class to keep your heart and lungs healthy. It may be as simple as walking for half an hour a day, doing a water exercise class, or doing household chores. Anything that gets you moving counts toward your daily exercise.

Arthritis patients should do some kind of cardiovascular exercise at least four days a week. One day of the week, that might mean doing household chores and walking for ten minutes to pick up something at the store. Another day, it might mean taking a half-hour walk or bicycle ride, swimming, or attending an exercise class. Mix and match activities you enjoy. Remember that the longer you go without movement, the harder it will be to get going when you finally get around to it.

If you have significant pain and stiffness in your joints, you may find that adding extra activity into your day wherever you can is the most comfortable approach. This may simply mean parking at the far end of the lot and walking, or walking on an errand rather than driving. While it's important to get your heart pumping, it's also important to listen to the messages your body is sending you. If the pain is severe, back off and rest. There's always tomorrow.

If you have arthritis in your hips, knees, or ankles, you may not be able to do weight-bearing exercise such as walking or aerobic dance. Your safest options under those circumstances are bicycling, swimming, or water aerobics. Stationary bicycling is a good alternative, because the level of resistance can be changed to match your tolerance from day to day. Swimming and water aerobics are great choices for arthritis, especially for those who are overweight.

Don't worry about measuring your heart rate. Focus instead on how you are feeling. If you are breathing deeply and quickly and are breaking a sweat, you're working hard enough. Try having a conversation with someone while you're exercising. If you can't speak a sentence a few words long without taking a breath, back off a little. If your joint pain is restricting you from working this hard, don't worry about it—just keep moving. Even if all you can do is work joints through their ranges of motion (see the next section for more on this), it's better than doing nothing.

Warm Up First

It's important to warm up your joints before doing cardiovascular exercise. Doing your range-of-motion exercises first (see pages 100–106) is a good way to accomplish this end. If you'd like to do something quicker, try the full-body warm-up routine below. Spending about five minutes on these exercises before doing your cardiovascular workout will help your joints become loose, warm, and more stable. Gently massaging joints that are especially stiff can help prepare you for exercise. Don't massage a joint that is hot and red.

You can also relieve stiffness with a hot shower or bath, or by applying a heating pad or hot water bottle. The application of heat increases blood flow and soothes away pain. If you tend to have significant pain during or after exercise, you may want to take your pain-relieving supplements before you start (see chapter 6). If your joints are inflamed, you're better off applying cold before exercise. Heat can make inflammation worse, while cold helps reduce swelling and pain. Apply an ice pack, an ice cube, or a bag of frozen peas to any inflamed joints. Remove the cold as soon as the area becomes numb; don't leave it on for more than twenty minutes. Wrapping the cold pack in a moist towel will help ease the chill. If you have any type of disorder that makes you sensitive to cold, such as vasculitis or Raynaud's phenomenon, don't apply ice. Check with your doctor or physical therapist for other options.

Full Body Warm-up Routine: This routine is also a good one for getting out of bed in the morning, when stiffness can be the worst.

1. Lie on your back on your bed or on the floor. Hug one knee into your chest at a time, then do some pedaling motions with your feet in the air.
2. Push your arms up toward the ceiling, fingers wide, and circle your wrists around a few times.
3. Hug both knees into your chest, then drop them to the right for a few breaths and to the left for a few more breaths.
4. Roll onto your belly and come up on all fours. Round your back up toward the ceiling like a cat, then arch it so that your belly drops toward the floor. Repeat several times. (If this hurts your wrists and hands, bend your elbows so that you're resting

on your forearms. Place some folded blankets or pillows beneath your forearms to bring your back flat.) Come to a seated position by dropping your hips to one side, and if you're on your bed scoot to the edge. If you're sitting on the floor, you may want to sit on a pillow or chair for exercises five through eight.

5. Tilt your head from side to side, drop your chin to your chest for a few breaths, then look back over each shoulder a few times.

6. Shrug your shoulders up and let them drop, then circle your shoulders back and forward a few times each.

7. Circle your arms as though you were swimming the crawl stroke, then circle them back as though you were doing the backstroke.

8. Bend and straighten your elbows.

9. Straighten your legs one at a time, circling your foot as you hold the leg straight. (If you are sitting on the floor, do this one lying on your back.)

After you finish your cardiovascular workout, be sure to do some stretching. The range of motion and flexibility exercises described in this chapter will stretch your joints without stressing them.

Water Exercise

Because it alleviates some of the stress of gravity on the joints, water exercise is ideal for those who have severe arthritis in weight-bearing joints (hips, knees, ankles, and feet). Lap swimming, water jogging, and treading water are all excellent cardiovascular exercises. Accessories for water exercise are easy to find in most sporting goods stores—for example, a foam flotation belt can be worn for water jogging, and foam "weights" can be used for resistance training in the water. Plastic hand paddles and swim fins can be helpful for those with arthritic feet and hands.

Any of the range of motion, flexibility, and strengthening exercises described in this chapter can be done in the water. Many gyms, hospitals, and community pools offer water aerobics classes, where an instructor leads participants through cardiovascular and strengthening exercises in warm, shallow water, often to music. You can find water exercise classes for arthritis patients in your area by contacting your local branch of the Arthritis Foundation.

Flexibility and Range of Motion Exercises

This type of exercise is extremely important for people with arthritis. Even when you can't do any other exercise, do your best to keep up with these. Range of motion exercises are designed simply to move joints in the ways they are designed to move. Flexibility exercises are designed to increase the flexibility of the tendons, ligaments, and muscles around a joint. The exercises below are a combination of both. Moving your joints—whether you do so in daily activities, or by doing flexibility and range of motion exercises—is the only way to preserve their function.

Try to push the movement of the joint as far as it will go without severe pain. Go a tiny bit beyond your comfort zone. Use your breath to help you stretch, by relaxing further into each stretch as you exhale. When you hit a place in an exercise that hurts or is extremely stiff, pause there for a full breath, allowing the exhalation to relax your joint through the sticky part. Resist the urge to tighten up.

Here are some range of motion and flexibility exercises for you to try. Focus on the ones for the joints that give you the most difficulty. Repeat each exercise three to eight times, moving slowly and steadily, breathing deeply, and resting between repetitions if necessary. Do the whole series twice each day. You might try doing them right after breakfast and right after dinner. If you're strapped for time, focus on the exercises for joints you have particular trouble with.

Once you learn them, you can do them anytime: waiting in line at the bank, sitting at a traffic light, or while watching TV or talking on the phone. The more often you do them, the easier they will get.

For Your Fingers

Finger Extender: Place one palm on a table and press the hand flat with the other hand.

Finger to Palm Stretch: Curl each finger toward your palm, one at a time, trying to touch the fingertips to the palm. Use your other hand to increase the distance each finger will stretch.

Thumb Touches: Touch each fingertip in succession to the tip of the thumb, stretching your fingers and thumb straight in between.

For Your Wrists

Inner Wrist Stretch: Press your palms together, slightly intertwining your fingertips. Use one hand at a time to press the other hand back, stretching the inner wrist.

Back of Wrist Stretch: Hang one hand over the edge of a table, palm down, and use the other hand to press the fingers toward the floor, stretching the back side of the wrist.

Wrist Twists: Place both forearms on a table, palms down. Without lifting the elbows, turn the palms up, then turn them back down.

Elbows

Across-the-Body Chop: Press palms together and touch them to your right shoulder. Extend the arms straight across your body, touching the hands to the outside of the left knee (if seated) or the outside of the left hip (if standing). Work to get the elbows as straight as possible. After three to eight repetitions, reverse it.

Shoulders and Chest

Shoulder Circles: Roll the shoulders forward, up, back, and down. Make the circles large and slow.

Shoulder Pivot: Hold your upper arm against your side, elbow at a right angle, forearm pointing forward, and palm facing inward. Take your wrist sideways, until the palm faces front and the forearm points directly to the side. Keep your upper arm against your side throughout.

Shoulder Opener: Clasp your hands at the base of your skull, press your elbows back, and then bring the elbows toward one another in front of your face.

Elbow Clasp: Reach both hands behind you and grasp each wrist in the other hand. Keep your shoulders down and your chest broad. If this is comfortable, begin to walk your hands up your forearms, aiming to clasp your elbows.

Over-the-Head: Hold a light stick (or a scarf or rope drawn taut) at either end, at about chest level. There should be a distance of two to three feet between your hands. Raise the stick or scarf overhead, then return to chest level. If you can pass it completely over your head and down your back, go ahead and do so.

Shoulder Pulley: Toss a rope over the top of an open door, then stand with your back to the edge of the door. Grab an end of the rope in each hand, pulling down on one end at a time so that the other hand gets pulled overhead.

Hips

Lying Twist: Lying on your back with knees bent, cross your right knee over the top of your left. Allow both legs to drop to the right, trying to ease them to the floor. Hold the stretch for up to one minute, then do the other side, crossing the left knee over the right and letting the legs fall to the left.

Knee Hug: Lying on your back, hug one knee at a time into the chest. You can keep the other leg bent with the foot on the floor, or extend it straight. Hold the stretch for up to a minute before switching sides.

Hip Opener: Start this one lying on your back with both knees bent, feet on the floor. Cross the right ankle just above the left knee, trying to point the right knee out to the side. Your right leg should form a triangle with your left thigh. If this feels easy, you can reach for your legs and bring them toward your chest. Hold for up to a minute. Don't do this one if you have had a hip replacement.

Side Leg Scissor: Lie on your back with your legs together and knees straight. Open your legs as wide as possible, then bring them back together.

Back Leg Extension: Stand facing a wall or chair, holding on for balance. Extend one leg straight back, keeping both legs straight and your hips square. (Imagine your hipbones have headlights in them, and you want to shine them straight ahead.) You can also do this one lying on your belly.

Boot Scoot: Sit in a straight-backed chair, with your hips all the way back in the seat. Scoot forward on the bones in your buttocks, moving one hip forward at a time, until you reach the front edge of the chair, and then scoot back.

Knees

Knee Bending: Sit on the edge of a straight-backed chair and walk one foot as far beneath the chair as it will go, trying to bend the knee as much as possible. Hold for up to one minute.

Knee Straightening: Sit on a chair and place one leg on a footstool. Use the muscles in the front of the thigh to try to straighten the knee completely. If this feels easy, try leaning over the extended leg, keeping your back flat. You'll feel a powerful stretch in the back of the thigh. Hold for up to one minute.

Ankles

Stair Stretch: Stand on a stair where a wall or railing is within easy reach. Turn so that your heels are at the edge of the stair, toes pointing away from the edge. Scoot the right heel back behind the left so that it hangs off the edge of the step, the ball of the foot still firmly planted. Bend the left knee, keeping the right knee straight. The right heel will press down below the level of the step, stretching the right calf muscle and ankle. Hold for up to one minute, then switch sides.

Happy Feet: Sit in a straight-backed chair, feet firmly on the floor. Lift your toes toward your nose, then lift your heels so that the balls of your feet and your toes are pressing into the floor. Try walking the feet to the right using this motion, then back to the left. Repeat three to eight times.

Ankle Circles: Sit in a chair and extend both legs forward slightly, so that the feet are off the floor. Draw big circles with your toes, both clockwise and counterclockwise.

Rolling Feet: Place a dowel on the floor in front of your chair (a broom handle or rolling pin should work fine, too), so that you can place the arches of your feet on it. Roll the feet front and back to stretch and massage your arches.

Neck

Half Head Rolls: Drop your right ear toward your right shoulder, without lifting the shoulder toward the ear. Then, drop your chin down toward your chest and roll your head to the left side, dropping the ear toward the shoulder. Repeat, rolling the head back to the right, four to eight times.

Head Turning: Turn your head to look over each of your shoulders. Inhale first, then turn the head slowly through the exhale. Inhale as you return your head to the center. Repeat two to four times per side.

Back

Stomach Crunches: Lie on your back, knees bent, feet elevated on the seat of a chair. Use your abdominal muscles to raise your hips and press your lower back into the floor. This is a very small movement and can be hard to master. You can try having a friend put his or her hand beneath the small of your back, so that you can feel as though you are pressing on something.

Knee Hug: Hug one knee at a time to the chest, or hug in both knees at once.

The Cobra: Lie on your belly and place your palms flat on the ground beside your shoulders. Keeping your elbows on the floor, press your head and chest up, gently arching your back. Drop your shoulders away from your ears and don't clench your buttocks. Look straight ahead.

Elbow Touch: Sit or stand and try to touch your elbows together behind you.

Cat Stretch: On all fours, arch your back toward the ceiling, then stretch the opposite way, so that your belly drops toward the ground.

Strengthening Exercise

Strength training, also known as *resistance training,* involves pitting a muscle against some type of resistance. Going to the gym and pumping iron is resistance training. So is holding on to the back of a chair and exercising the leg muscles by squatting partway down and rising. Pushing and pulling a vacuum cleaner also qualifies. At the gym, the weights provide resistance; in the case of the squats, the weight of the body provides resistance; with the vacuuming, of course, it's the vacuum.

It's important to do some kind of resistance training. Muscle and tendon strength quickly disappear if they aren't challenged regularly. Resistance training also stimulates the bones to build themselves up. Weight-bearing exercise (walking or jogging) is universally recommended because of its bone-building effects, and it's especially important for those who can't do weight-bearing exercise to stick to a thorough strengthening program.

Don't think that being unable to hold on to weights or tubing because of arthritis makes you unable to do resistance training. There are plenty of options for you that use only your own body, the wall, or the floor as resistance. For some of the exercises described here, you can increase their intensity by using a belt, rope, inner tube, or surgical tubing. (Whatever you use should be about three feet long when laid out flat, so that it's about a foot and a half long doubled over.)

Many of the exercises recommended for strengthening fragile joints are *isometric exercises.* This means the joint is held in the same position as the muscle is tensed and released. If you were to press your palms together to work your arm muscles, you would be doing an isometric exer-

cise. Others move the joint through its range of motion
with gentle resistance.

These exercises are simple and easy to do at home,
without any expensive equipment. As you pull or push
into the resistance, exhale smoothly. Each repetition
should take you about three seconds. After a count of
three, relax the muscles long enough to take a deep inhalation, then repeat. Perform eight to fifteen repetitions
of each exercise, moving slowly and steadily. Do the se-
quence on three or four nonconsecutive days of the week.
If you don't have time to do the whole series, focus on the
ones for the joints that give you the most trouble.

Don't do any strengthening exercises involving any
joints that are red, hot, and swollen. Only perform the
range of motion and flexibility exercises for those joints
until the inflammation goes down.

Fingers, Hands, and Wrists

Ball Squeeze: Squeeze and release a rubber ball.

Finger to Thumb Press: Press the tip of each finger suc-
cessively against the tip of the thumb.

Finger Lift: Put the right hand palm down on a table and
place the left hand over the fingers. Lift and lower the fingers of the right hand, resisting their movement with the
left. Reverse.

Finger Scoot: This exercise is especially good for those
with rheumatoid arthritis, which often leads to a drifting
of the fingers toward the pinky-side of the hand. Lay one
hand flat on a table, fingers together and thumb spread

wide. Move each finger, one at a time, toward the thumb. Use your other hand to help if needed.

Wrist Lift: Place your right hand palm down on a table and place your left palm on top of it. Try to lift the right hand up from the wrist, providing resistance with the left, strengthening the top of the right wrist. Repeat with your other hand. Then, do the same exercise, but with the palm of the working hand facing up, to work the muscles on the inside of the wrist.

Shoulders, Chest, and Elbows

Door Jamb Push: Stand in a doorway with the backs of your wrists against the door jamb. Inhale, then press out steadily as you exhale for three counts, as though you were trying to raise your hands up past your ears. Inhale as you relax your arms.

Door Jamb Push, Part Two: Now, stand behind the doorway and reach both arms forward at shoulder level, palms facing each other. Press the arms away from one another.

Tug-of-War: Place your exercise belt around your wrists. With the upper arms against your sides and forearms pointing front, press one wrist down toward the floor and the other up toward the ceiling. Hold for a count of three, exhaling, and inhale as you release.

Tug-of-War, Part Two: Try the same exercise with the arms extended straight in front of you. You'll feel this one more in the shoulders.

Bow and Arrow: Hold your exercise belt as though you were holding a bow and arrow. Pull the hands in opposite directions, exhaling as you pull and inhaling as you release. Repeat to the other side.

Prayer Press: Put your palms together in front of your chest as though you were praying. Inhale, then press the palms together steadily as you exhale.

Hips and Buttocks

Squeeze and Release: Sitting in a chair with your feet on the floor, squeeze your knees together, then open them slightly. If you have a soft exercise ball for hand exercises, you can squeeze it between your knees.

Side Leg Press: Sit in a chair with your exercise belt around both legs, just below the knees. Tie it so that it's taut when the knees are six to eight inches apart. Inhale, then press your knees away from each other through the exhale.

Knees and Ankles

Leg Straightener: Sit in a chair and extend one leg straight in front of you at a time, holding for a count of three before slowly releasing it down.

Leg Bending: Stand and hold on to something for balance, feet about four inches apart. Bend one knee, bringing the heel toward the buttock, trying to keep the thighs together. Actively tuck your hips under as you do this, to avoid straining your back.

Ankle and Foot Strengthener: Stand with your feet four to six inches apart. Hold on to a chair or the wall if needed. Rise slowly onto your tiptoes and lower down just as slowly.

Neck

Head Lift: Lie on your back with your head on a pillow. Lift your head up, bringing your chin toward your chest.

Head Press: Press the back of your head into the pillow.

Stomach and Back

Stomach Crunches: see page 106.

Back Press: Sit on the floor and lean your back against a wall. Press your back into the wall for counts of three.

Bow Pose: Lie on your belly on a soft surface, with your forehead on the floor, arms by your sides, and legs straight. Inhale, and as you exhale gently raise your head, shoulders, and legs off the ground. Look toward the floor to avoid straining your neck. (Don't do this exercise if you are having low back pain.)

Training Your Balance Muscles

It's common for people to have trouble keeping their balance as they age. Falls that barely scratch a young person can seriously harm an older person, whose reflexes are slow to kick in. Doing balance exercises is an important part of preventing falls and preserving your sense of safety in your day-to-day activities. In fact, it isn't getting older that makes us lose our ability to balance as much as it is the lack of physical activity that usually goes along with aging. The Asian disciplines of Tai Chi, Chi Gong, and yoga are an excellent way to preserve balance, and classes are readily available in most urban and suburban areas. You'll find out more about them in the next section.

Some of the exercises already described are excellent for balance training. Here are a few others to add to your routine:

Walk the Line: Walk heel-to-toe along a straight line on the ground. A crack along the pavement will do, or any other straight line you can find to follow. If your balance is very poor, don't try to go heel-to-toe right away; just try to walk the line until that becomes comfortable.

One-Footed Balance: Stand near a chair or wall that you can grab if you lose your balance. Raise one foot just off the ground and balance on the other foot. If you can't do this without hanging on, try using your hand lightly to hold on, without leaning your weight onto it.

Other Kinds of Exercise for Arthritis

Traditional exercise forms such as yoga, Tai Chi, and Chi Gong are wonderful for the joints. They all share common characteristics: each promotes strength, balance, and coordination; and all incorporate the use of the breath. These disciplines are often called "enlightened exercise."

Yoga originated in India, and has been practiced in many different forms for thousands of years. It combines attention to proper alignment with deep stretches and standing poses to strengthen the large muscle groups of the lower body. Poses are held for several breaths. If you have arthritis, take a gentle class where you will receive plenty of attention from the instructor. There are alternate poses that can be substituted for those that hurt arthritic joints, so don't hesitate to ask the instructor for alternatives during class. Yoga classes often include meditation and end with a period of total relaxation.

Tai Chi is an Oriental martial art form. Its slow, dance-like movements are based on patterns in nature. There are actually many different kinds of Tai Chi, some of which are more challenging than others. Look for a class geared toward older people if you have arthritis. The exercises are performed from a standing position and involve a great deal of weight-shifting, turning, and pivoting on the feet, with expansive arm gestures.

Chi Gong, or qigong, is also an Oriental practice. (Chi Gong is an Anglicized spelling of the Chinese name, which translates more closely to *qigong*—different spelling, same pronunciation.) More than 60 million people practice qigong daily in China. It is not only a form of exercise, but also a form of meditation and a self-healing practice. Posture, breathing, and mental focus are all part of Chi Gong exercises.

If you are interested in trying any of these practices, you will need to seek out the guidance of a teacher in your area. Classes in all three of these practices are available in most areas of the country. Try to find an experienced teacher who can help you adapt exercises to your needs. You may find that doing one of these practices gives you all the range-of-motion and flexibility exercise you need— and other gifts you won't expect.

Arthritis Exercise Programs

PACE (People with Arthritis Can Exercise) classes are offered by the Arthritis Foundation nationwide. They usually involve seated and standing exercises and are taught by qualified instructors. Contact the Arthritis Foundation in your area to find out where you can attend these classes. Exercise videos for home use are also available from the Arthritis Foundation. Call them at (800) 283-7800 for information or to order.

There are many books that go into greater depth on the topic of exercise for arthritis. Check your local bookstore if you feel you'd like more information on the subject. If you're undergoing physical therapy or occupational therapy, your therapist should be able to recommend good titles to you.

Nutritional Supplements
for Pain-Free Joints

The practice of treating disease with vitamin and mineral supplements, known as *orthomolecular medicine,* began in earnest with two-time Nobel laureate Linus Pauling's groundbreaking research on vitamin C in the late 1960s and 1970s. He found vitamin C to be a valuable treatment for the common cold, and also found that high doses of the vitamin dramatically prolonged the lives of terminal cancer patients. Since Dr. Pauling proposed the use of high doses of vitamins and minerals for the prevention and treatment of disease, an entire community of researchers and health practitioners has followed suit.

Today, naturopaths and complementary medicine physicians commonly prescribe supplemental nutrients to treat illness. This is not because they work as "magic bullets," but because they support and strengthen the body in ways that naturally bring us back to health. Due to the successes achieved with the orthomolecular approach, re-

search efforts in this area have expanded. The science behind it has led to better acceptance of orthomolecular
therapies by conventional medicine and literally thousands of scientific studies show the benefits of these types
of approaches.

When you make the decision to use nutritional supplements to treat a disease, your expectations may need a
little adjustment. After all, we've been led to believe that
every disease treatment should work fast to eliminate uncomfortable symptoms. When you use nutrients, the beneficial effects appear gradually and with more subtlety as
your body's healing systems are gently stimulated and
supported. It can take months to notice a difference, even
when you are religiously following your supplement plan.
Sometimes, results are quick and dramatic. If they aren't,
remember—it took you years to create this disease, so give
your body some time to heal.

Antioxidants and Free Radicals

Free radicals are submicroscopic particles that can cause
damage to cells. They are formed in the process of normal
metabolism, as cells transform protein, carbohydrate, and
fats into energy. They are also formed for specific jobs; for
example, the immune system creates free radicals to help
with the job of warding off infectious disease. Free radicals
are plentifully created during the process of inflammation,
and they are thought to play a significant role in both
rheumatoid and osteoarthritis.

The process of forming free radicals is called *oxidation.*
When an apple cut in half turns brown, that's oxidation.
Rusting metal is also oxidizing, and so is your skin when
you go out and fall asleep in a chair in the sun for too long.

Antioxidant nutrients are our natural defense against

free radicals. If antioxidants are readily available in the body, free radicals shouldn't build up enough to do any appreciable damage. Once the antioxidant has quenched a free radical, it becomes a free radical itself and needs to be replenished by another antioxidant. Different antioxidants have different "specialties." Some target the free radicals formed when fats are oxidized; others protect the liver from oxidation; others are especially good at replenishing other antioxidants. That's why it's so important to get a full spectrum of antioxidant nutrients—C, E, and beta-carotene especially—in adequate amounts.

The foods richest in antioxidant nutrients are vegetables and fruits. Most antioxidant supplements are derived from these foods. Humans also make *endogenous* antioxidants, including *glutathione* and *superoxide dismutase* (SOD). These antioxidants aren't found in foods, but nutrients found in foods and supplements—including zinc, copper, and sulfur—are needed to make the endogenous antioxidants.

Vitamin C

Research has shown that elderly people with cartilage disorders are usually deficient in vitamin C. This vitamin is needed to make collagen, the basic building block of all connective tissues. In studies on both animals and humans, high intakes of vitamin C reduced joint inflammation, decreased the rate of cartilage deterioration, and reduced the likelihood of joint pain. This vitamin appears also to stimulate the growth of cartilage and the production of anti-inflammatory prostaglandins.

Vitamin C is acidic, and high doses can cause stomach upset or diarrhea. If this is a concern for you, use a buffered version, such as calcium ascorbate or magnesium ascorbate. The cheapest way to buy vitamin C is as a powder, which you can stir into juice. Chewable vitamin C can damage tooth enamel. Also, consult your doctor about using high doses (over 500 mg/day) of vitamin C if you are taking diabetes medications. Too much C can counteract the effects of the medicine. Use from 1,000 to 3,000 mg a day in divided doses.

Quercetin

This antioxidant is part of a family of plant compounds called *bioflavonoids*. Bioflavonoids were once thought to simply increase the absorption of vitamin C. Now we know that the bioflavonoid nutrients are powerful antioxidants on their own and have great value in the treatment and prevention of inflammatory diseases. Quercetin, for example, suppresses inflammation in joints affected by RA, essentially by breaking the chain of events that causes the inflammatory process to balloon out of control. Those with osteoarthritis will benefit from quercetin's potency as an antioxidant.

Products containing both quercetin and bromelain (a protein-digesting enzyme, which is discussed in a few pages) are available. Try one that gives you 500 mg each of bromelain and quercetin. Use it twice a day.

Oligomeric Proanthocyanidins (OPCs)

Cranberries, bilberries, blueberries, blackberries, cherries, and purple grapes are examples of fruits that are rich in these plant pigments. Grape-seed extract also contains them. OPC supplements are also made from French maritime pine-tree bark, sold under the brand name Pycnogenol. The OPCs are incredibly powerful antioxidants. They readily donate electrons to oxidized vitamin C, reactivating it. On their own, they have been shown to have eighteen times the effectiveness of vitamin C and fifty times the effectiveness of vitamin E at neutralizing free radicals.

In RA and osteoarthritis, newly formed collagen tends to be abnormally stiff and prone to injury, with too many cross-linkages. Research has shown that OPCs promote the normal cross-linking of collagen.

The process of inflammation causes enzymes called *collagenases* to form. As the name implies, collagenases digest collagen. In healthy joints, collagenases perform a valuable function, clearing away old, damaged collagen to make room for new. In arthritic joints, collagenases appear to get carried away, digesting more than the body can replace. OPCs guard collagen from excessive collagenase activity.

Grape-seed extract is an excellent, inexpensive source of OPCs. Try taking 200 mg a day for two weeks, then a maintenance dose of 25 to 50 mg a day. Eat ripe red grapes, blueberries, and cherries (organic, please!), and enjoy a glass of red wine or red grape juice now and then. Both are rich sources of OPCs.

Vitamin E

Studies have shown that vitamin E has painkilling effects comparable to NSAIDs. Vitamin E is also the body's primary *fat-soluble* antioxidant. This means that it protects cell membranes (which are composed of fats) and the fats in the blood, such as cholesterol and triglycerides, from oxidation. The synovial membrane, which is the starting place of rheumatoid arthritis inflammation, is also made up of fats, and supplying enough vitamin E is thought to protect the synovium from free radical damage during inflammation. Early studies, performed in the 1960s, showed the potential of vitamin E to ease osteoarthritis symptoms.

Be aware that vitamin E is a blood thinner, and caution should be used if you are planning to have surgery—especially if you also happen to be taking blood-thinning medications or aspirin. If you are using either of these medications, or if you have a deficiency in the blood-clotting vitamin K, consult your health care provider before taking supplemental vitamin E. Anyone with an overactive thyroid (Graves' disease), high blood pressure, diabetes, or rheumatic heart disease should build up their vitamin E dose slowly, starting with 50 to 100 IU and adding 100 IU each month until 400 to 800 IU are taken daily.

Taking 400 to 800 IU of natural vitamin E, also called d-alpha tocopherol. (Synthetic is *dl*-alpha tocopherol; please don't use it.) Vitamin E is recommended for every adult. For anti-inflammatory effects, up to 1200 IU a day have been used, but you should not use more than 800 IU a day without a doctor's guidance.

Vitamin A and the Carotenes

Vitamin A, found in fish, butter, milk, and organ meats, is available in supplement form. Vitamin A stimulates the immune system and can be a powerful ally in fending off infections and healing infections and wounds. High doses of vitamin A—more than 50,000 IU per day for more than a week or two—can lead to toxicity. Women who are pregnant or may become pregnant should not use more than 15,000 IU of vitamin A per day. However, doses of 10,000 to 15,000 IU a day are quite safe and are an important part of every adult and child vitamin regimen.

Low levels of vitamin A and beta-carotene, a nutritional percursor of vitamin A, increase risk of autoimmune diseases in general. In most people, beta-carotene can be turned into vitamin A once it's in the body, but it also has many functions of its own.

Beta-carotene is one of about 600 carotenes. The carotenes are plant pigments, found plentifully in bright yellow and orange vegetables and fruits, some of which can be transformed into vitamin A in the body. The antioxidant activity of the carotenes is much greater than that of vitamin A. Beta-carotene is the best known of the carotenes and is most easily transformed to vitamin A, but there are at least thirty different carotenes that can undergo the conversion.

A mixed carotenoid supplement, including beta-carotene, lycopene, alpha-carotene, gamma-carotene, lutein, and zeaxanthin, will lend antioxidant support to arthritic joints. Eating plenty of brightly colored vegetables and fruits will also increase your carotene intake.

Vitamin D

This vitamin is needed for proper absorption of calcium and the building of healthy bones and cartilage. Damage to bones and cartilage is an end result of both RA and osteoarthritis, and low vitamin D levels have been found in people with arthritic diseases. In some research circles, it's thought that a defective gene may alter the action of vitamin D in the body, increasing the likelihood that those with the defect will end up with arthritis. Problems with vitamin D activity affect the cells that make cartilage and bone in joints affected by both types of arthritis, increasing the rate at which bone is broken down there. Vitamin D supplementation is an important preventative measure against osteoporosis.

If you are using fish liver oil supplements, check to see how much vitamin D they contain—you don't want to get too much. Vitamin D is a fat-soluble vitamin and can build up in the body to toxic levels. (Excess water-soluble vitamins are simply flushed away in the urine, while fat-soluble vitamins are stored away.)

Most adults under fifty should supplement 400 IU a day, and those over fifty should take 800 IU a day. If you get a daily dose of sunshine you can probably get by on 400 IU.

Niacin

The B vitamin niacin has been used in orthomolecular medicine to relieve RA and osteoarthritis symptoms since the 1950s. Very few clinical studies have been done to support its use for this purpose, but those that have been done have shown promising results. In one recent study, with 500 mg of niacin six times per day, joint mobility improved, and pain and the need for NSAIDs decreased. If you want to try high-dose niacin, start out by taking 50 mg of no-flush niacin (inositol hexaniacinate) three times a day with meals. You can gradually increase the dose up to 100 mg three times a day, but do so gradually, over the span of a month. Some people can tolerate as much as 300 mg daily, but this should only be taken under the supervision of a health care professional. Be sure to let your doctor know you are using niacin, especially if you have gout, stomach ulcers, liver disease, glaucoma, or severe diabetes.

Healthy Fats

Omega-3 fats (eicosapentaenoic acids, or EPAs).

You've already learned about the importance of getting plenty of EPAs in your diet. EPAs are the raw material from which anti-inflammatory eicosanoids are built. Low levels of EPAs have been found in the bodies of people with inflammatory diseases, and studies have shown that supplemental EPAs can help decrease autoimmune inflammation. Some of the subjects in the studies that back this therapy up were able to decrease their NSAID dosages with fish oil supplementation.

Most EPA supplements are derived from fish oils. The problem with fish oil supplements is that they go rancid—in other words, they oxidize—quite easily. Taking a rancid fish oil supplement is equivalent to swallowing a mouthful of free radicals, in which case the fish oil will do more harm than good. Even if you are able to protect it from heat and light and keep it in the refrigerator, it may have already become partly oxidized during processing. The recommended dose for treating RA symptoms is quite high—3 to 7 grams of fish oil a day (or 1.8 grams of EPA) for three to twelve months—and this can get expensive and be very unpleasant if it "burps" back up.

The best way to get your EPAs is by eating deepwater fish, and by cutting down on sources of fat that are transformed into pro-inflammatory eicosanoids—saturated fats from red meats and dairy products, hydrogenated fats, and vegetable oils. Your goal is to raise levels of omega-3s and decrease levels of pro-inflammatory fats. Whether you have osteoarthritis or rheumatoid arthritis, improving your balance of healthy fats in this way will improve your overall health.

For some people with rheumatoid arthritis, EPA supplementation with fish oil may be worth a try, because much higher doses of EPA can be concentrated in a capsule than can be obtained through the diet. Just be sure that it's well preserved. Break open a capsule and smell it—if it smells rancid (versus just fishy) find another brand.

Flaxseed oil

For raising omega-3 levels, some health experts recommend supplemental flaxseed oil over fish oil. Flax oil contains another type of omega-3 fatty acid, *alpha-linoleic acid* (ALA). In order to serve as raw material for the anti-inflammatory eicosanoids, ALA must be converted to EPA in the body. Flax oil supplementation doesn't raise blood levels of EPA as much as fish oil does. If you decrease your intake of polyunsaturated vegetable oils—that means safflower, sunflower, and corn oils, used in many high-fat processed foods—flax is more effective at raising the level of EPA. Another problem with flaxseed oil is that it is one of the most unstable oils in existence—so much so that by the time you get it home from the store, it's probably rancid.

One good bet for including flax in your anti-inflammatory regimen is to buy whole flaxseeds. Within the seed are antioxidant substances that protect the fats from becoming oxidized. You can grind them into a fine meal in a coffee grinder and sprinkle them onto salads, cereals, and soups. Keep the seeds in the refrigerator. Buy only small amounts at a time, and grind them only as needed. This is an excellent way to add nutritious, fiber-rich whole seeds to your diet.

Please don't use too much flax oil, or it could have the opposite effect you intended, increasing the free radical load in the body. Remember, Mother Nature has seen fit to package these types of oils in very small amounts, mainly in vegetables, nuts, seeds, and whole grains. In tiny amounts they're much needed, but in high amounts they can be destructive. The imbalance of fats and oils found in North American culture is caused more by an *excess* of saturated fats and hydrogenated oils, and virtually none of the other types of oils. The idea is to strive for balance. If you cut out hydrogenated oils altogether and eat a moderate amount of saturated fat and monounsaturated oils and plenty of fresh vegetables, nuts, seeds, whole grains, and fish, your fatty acid balance should be fine.

Omega-6 Fats

These fats are rich in *gamma-linoleic acid,* or GLA. They are found in safflower, sunflower, and soybean oils, and are also sold as supplements made from evening primrose, black currant, or borage oils. Omega-6 fats can be transformed into either "good" or "bad" eicosanoids, depending on the presence of certain enzymes. Because it isn't known exactly how to ensure that omega-6 fats go into making good eicosanoids, there is some controversy around its use in the treatment of rheumatoid arthritis.

Studies on rheumatoid arthritis patients lasting up to one year have shown significant improvements in pain, swelling, morning stiffness, and the number of tender and swollen joints with very high supplemental doses of GLA. Results of GLA studies haven't been consistent, however, and it has been shown that long-term supplementation of omega-6 oils can lead to decreases in levels of EPA (the fats that turn into "good" eicosanoids) and increases in levels of arachidonic acid (the fats that turn into "bad" eicosanoids). Most people get plenty of omega-6 oils in the form of vegetable oils and don't need additional GLA.

Enzymes

Supplementation of dietary enzymes, which are a part of all fresh plant foods, is often beneficial to people with rheumatoid arthritis. They are thought to work by slowing down inflammatory reactions themselves, and by activating immune cells that do the same. There is some scientific evidence in favor of dietary enzyme therapy for rheumatoid arthritis. Pain from muscle injuries, which usually involves inflammation, has also been shown to respond well to bromelain.

Many people find that 100 to 500 mg of bromelain (a protein-digesting enzyme derived from pineapple) three times a day between meals improves their mobility and decreases their joint swelling. Protein-digesting enzymes seem to work best. Pancreatin, papain, and trypsin are other protein-digesting enzymes you might want to try. If you find that the enzymes make you nauseated, try taking them with meals instead of between meals. Once you stop taking it, symptoms that were relieved by the enzyme supplement are likely to return—so if it works for you, keep using it. Supplements that contain 500 mg bromelain and 500 mg quercetin per dose are ideal.

MSM

Methylsulfonylmethane, or MSM, is one of the most exciting nutritional supplements available for the treatment of rheumatoid and osteoarthritis symptoms. The potential uses of MSM are many: it relieves pain and inflammation, improves blood flow by dilating blood vessels, reduces formation of scar tissue, improves health of skin, hair, and nails, helps normalize the immune system, reduces muscle spasm, and even has some anti-parasite activity.

Ever soaked in a hot sulfur spring? If you have, you know how soothing it can be. For centuries, people have sought out sulfur springs because of their healing effect on arthritic diseases, skin conditions, and even digestive disorders. MSM contains organic sulfur—the form in which the mineral sulfur occurs in living cells.

Early in the history of the therapeutic use of sulfur, another form, called DMSO, was used to treat painful joints and inflammatory diseases with notable success. The problem with DMSO was its side effects, which included a distinct garlicky odor, rash, nasal congestion, breathlessness, and allergic reactions. These side effects were bad enough to cause scientists to lose interest in researching DMSO as an arthritis remedy—that is, until the recent discovery that MSM was the main healing ingredient and could be isolated and used without these side effects.

MSM is thought to work against arthritis pain and inflammation by several different mechanisms:

- MSM donates sulfur molecules for the manufacture of collagen. (More specifically, sulfur is a component of *glucosamine,* which you'll learn about in depth in the next chapter.) Without adequate sulfur, the body can't repair the damage that happens naturally with daily wear and tear, or the accelerated damage seen in arthritis. As with many of the nutrients discussed in this chapter, sulfur levels tend to be low in people with arthritis.
- Sulfur is also a component of glutathione, the most important antioxidant made in the body. Low levels of glutathione mean decreased ability to quench free radicals that contribute to joint damage.
- It reduces muscle spasm around arthritic joints. Muscle spasm occurs in damaged joints as they try to protect themselves from further damage, and these knots can contribute a great deal to joint pain.
- MSM relieves inflammation. It is thought to have this effect due to a sensitizing effect, making the body more sensitive to its own anti-inflammatory hormones—particularly cortisol. When patients use

sulfur derivatives such as DMSO and MSM, their
need for cortisone drugs (synthetic pharmaceutical
versions of cortisol) drops. In uncontrolled inflammation, fibroblasts (which manufacture connective
tissues) work overtime, making tissues that don't
function properly. DMSO, and possibly MSM, also
slow down swelling and scar tissue formation by reducing the activity of fibroblasts. Sulfur compounds
are also thought to remove excess fluid from sites of
inflammation.

- MSM relieves pain. No one knows exactly how, but
there are a few solid theories. It's been shown to inhibit the nerve impulses that send pain messages from
injured tissues to the brain. Reduction of inflammation and muscle spasm also reduce pain sensations.

MSM is available as a topical cream or gel, and in powder, capsule, and tablet forms. It's well absorbed through
the skin. Some proponents advise using it topically and
internally at the same time for increased effectiveness. It
appears that using glucosamine, which is discussed in detail in the next chapter, and MSM at the same time also
has increased healing effects on arthritis.

Recommended Dosage

The recommended oral dose is 1,800 to 9,000 milligrams
a day, divided into three doses with meals. Start with the
lowest dose and work up slowly, adding 300 mg each time
you increase the dose. For some people, MSM works right
away, and for others it takes a few weeks. The only side effects you might encounter are mild gastrointestinal upset
or diarrhea. If you tend to be constipated, MSM may be
just the thing for you—one of its perks is that it relieves
constipation.

Natural Remedies
for Arthritis Symptoms

Nature is rich with substances that have potent healing powers. In the age of high-tech medicine, natural remedies are often looked upon as primitive and rudimentary—definitely not a match for the designer chemicals commonly known as drugs. The truth is that Mother Nature is far more intelligent a healer than any scientist puttering away in a laboratory. Research is beginning to reveal exactly how time-tested natural remedies work to restore balanced good health.

In this chapter, you'll find out more about natural remedies that can relieve osteoarthritis and rheumatoid arthritis symptoms. Some work by the same mechanisms as prescription drugs, while others have unique modes of action to repair damaged cartilage and counter inflammation.

There are many natural healing options for people with arthritis. Don't be daunted by the sheer number of them.

They aren't meant to be tried all at once. Some are specific for rheumatoid arthritis, osteoarthritis, or both, so that should help you to narrow down your choices. Start minimally, with one or two natural remedies, and build up from there. Allow a few weeks for each to begin to work.

Help for Damaged Cartilage

Glucosamine Sulfate (Osteoarthritis)

Many of the supplements and natural remedies described in this book are designed to decrease inflammation, which is most often a characteristic of rheumatoid arthritis. Osteoarthritis symptoms may not respond as well to anti-inflammatory measures. Damaged cartilage, not inflammation, is the reason for osteoarthritis pain and disability. Any cure for osteoarthritis would have to give the body the means to repair cartilage.

Glucosamine (glue-KOH-suh-meen) *sulfate* does just that. This cartilage-supporting therapy for osteoarthritis is backed up by scientific studies performed in the United States and abroad. Glucosamine sulfate is significantly more effective than placebo (sugar pill) at relieving osteoarthritis pain, stiffness, and swelling, and it is just as effective as NSAIDs at achieving these ends. It does this without any of NSAIDs' harmful effects on the digestive tract and without causing further deterioration of cartilage. Despite this evidence, many conventional physicians continue to deny its potential usefulness in the treatment of osteoarthritis.

Glucosamine is derived from animal cartilage. It belongs to a family of substances called *glycosaminoglycans* (GAGs)—sugars and proteins bound together. These GAG molecules link together to form *proteoglycans* (PGs). Proteoglycans, in turn, link to form connective tissue, weaving through the gridwork of collagen fibers. PGs are also needed to make the synovial fluid that lubricates and cushions joints.

In growing children, glucosamine and other GAGs (about 50 percent of GAGs in cartilage are glucosamine) are manufactured at a rapid clip. Throughout childhood and young adulthood, new GAGs are made as rapidly as they are worn out. In other words, in a young body, the turnover of connective tissue substances is rapid, and this keeps the joints springy and flexible. With aging, GAG production falls dramatically, and the deterioration of GAGs begins to surpass their renewal. Cartilage becomes less resilient and more easily worn down with wear and tear.

When researchers look at arthritic cartilage under a microscope, the proteoglycan chains appear worn, frayed, and shrunken in size compared to those seen in healthy cartilage. There is also less water stored in arthritic cartilage. Without an adequate fluid cushion, cartilage becomes less resilient and more vulnerable to the damaging effects of friction.

A shortage of glucosamine slows down production of GAGs and PGs, and the logic of glucosamine supplementation is to give the body what it needs to build these protein-sugar molecules. Since the early 1980s, many meticulously performed studies have shown that glucosamine supplements do in fact decrease pain and improve mobility. They don't ultimately destroy more cartilage, as NSAIDs do, but make the building blocks of cartilage available so that the body can actually heal the joints.

Making a biochemical building block available to the body doesn't always mean that it goes to where it's needed and is properly utilized. In the case of glucosamine sulfate, it not only goes to where it's needed—it actually stimulates the formation of new cartilage. Glucosamine sulfate also stimulates the production of *hyaluronic acid* in synovial fluid, which keeps the fluid viscous and gives it its shock-absorbing quality. As if all of these therapeutic effects weren't enough to recommend it, glucosamine is also a mild anti-inflammatory.

Glucosamine sulfate is very well absorbed through the GI tract. The only adverse effects reported have been mild GI discomfort, drowsiness, skin reactions, and headache, but they are rarely severe enough to cause people to stop using it.

Anyone with osteoarthritis should give glucosamine sulfate a try. Buy a reputable brand, because there are a lot of less-than-ethical manufacturers jumping on the bandwagon and selling inferior supplements. Use 1,500 mg a day in divided doses. When used with MSM and antioxidants, it is even more effective at slowing the progress of, or even reversing, the course of osteoarthritis.

Chondroitin Sulfate (Osteoarthritis)

Many advocates of glucosamine advise osteoarthritis patients to also use *chondroitin sulfate*. Chondroitin is another element of cartilage. It is made up of various glycosaminoglycans (GAGs), including glucosamine sulfate. Under a microscope, chondroitin is seen as short branches coming off of the pine-tree–like proteoglycan (PG) molecules. In cartilage, chondroitin and glucosamine have the same relationship as magnets turned the wrong way— they repel one another. This creates open spaces within the cartilage, which act like the open spaces in a sponge: when you squeeze the sponge, water is forced out, but as soon as you release your grip the water returns. This is how cartilage maintains its springiness.

In aging cartilage, chondroitin sulfate chains become smaller, and less water is drawn in. Researchers have attempted to show that supplemental chondroitin would add to the positive effects of glucosamine on arthritic joints, and the results of their studies have been positive but not conclusive. A few studies have shown positive results with chondroitin alone, but most of them were performed with injected rather than oral chondroitin. This large molecule is not at all well absorbed in the GI tract, and is much more expensive than glucosamine. Try glucosamine alone for six to eight weeks. If it doesn't have the effects you were hoping for, try a supplement that will give you 1,500 mg of glucosamine and 1,200 mg of chondroitin a day.

Ginger Extract (Rheumatoid Arthritis and Osteoarthritis)

Ginger is more than a pungent, delicious spice. It's a natural remedy that has been used for more than 5,000 years to treat digestive problems and pain. In Ayurvedic medicine, ginger is part of so many herbal formulations that it is known as *vishwabhesaj,* or "universal medicine." The root, or *rhizome,* of the ginger plant contains a sticky resin packed with over 400 different biochemicals.

Scientists have isolated and tested these chemicals to discover what gives ginger its healing powers, and it turns out that several of them are natural inhibitors of the formation of "bad" pro-inflammatory eicosanoids. Dr. Morton Weidner, a Danish biochemist, spent six years in his quest to create a natural arthritis remedy from a special Chinese strain of ginger. He isolated the active constituents and painstakingly tested them in his laboratory, trying to discover what combination of these constituents would most effectively reduce pain and inflammation from osteoarthritis and rheumatoid arthritis. His quest led to the formulation of an extract he called EV.EXT 33. A faster-acting version, called EV.EXT 77, has since been developed.

This ginger extract works to soothe arthritis symptoms through several mechanisms. It inhibits the formation of pro-inflammatory prostaglandins by about 20 percent, making it a natural COX-2 inhibitor. Unlike any of the drugs available for arthritis, EV.EXT 33 effectively prevents the production of pro-inflammatory *leukotrienes*— eicosanoids that play a major role in the inflammatory process. Dr. Weidner's research showed that while the COX enzymes played a role in short-term joint discomfort, the lipoxygenase enzymes (which lead to the formation of "bad" leukotrienes) are more instrumental in creating long-term joint discomfort. Because it suppresses both COX-2 and lipoxygenase, it is known as a *dual inhibitor.* Ginger extract also acts as an antioxidant, calming the burst of free radicals formed when inflammation strikes.

This special herbal formulation also suppresses the formation of an immune system component called *tumor necrosis factor-alpha* (TNF-alpha). TNF-alpha's job is to summon other biochemicals that stimulate sensations of pain and eat away at collagen fibers. Levels of TNF-alpha are higher in the joints of osteoarthritis patients than in normal joints. When an arthritic joint is stressed repeatedly it releases TNF-alpha into the body in large quantities. Suppressing it reduces pain, inflammation, and joint damage. EV.EXT 33 also encourages the formation of biochemicals responsible for the rebuilding of joint tissues damaged by inflammation.

In some people, the extract works its magic within a month's time, and in others it may take a little longer.

Using fresh ginger root, powdered ginger, or whole ginger root supplements isn't going to have the same level of effectiveness against arthritis symptoms. There are over a hundred different species of ginger grown around the world, and each root's composition is different. A carefully standardized extract like EV.EXT 33, specially composed to work against arthritis symptoms, is a much better bet.

Herbal Extracts for Arthritis

Boswellin (Boswellia serrata, or Indian frankincense; rheumatoid arthritis): This 4,000-year-old Ayurvedic remedy relieves inflammation slightly better than the prescription NSAID phenylbutazone. It suppresses the production of pro-inflammatory eicosanoids and interrupts the chain of events that leads to out-of-control inflammation. The formation of inflammatory lipoxygenases is especially well controlled with boswellin. The therapeutic dose is 600 mg a day, in divided doses.

Cat's Claw or Una de Gato (Unicaria tomentosa; osteoarthritis and rheumatoid arthritis): Derived from the bark of a tree found in South America, cat's claw is a traditional Peruvian remedy for digestion problems and arthritis. It has antioxidant, anti-inflammatory, and immunity-modifying actions. It's especially useful for the treatment of osteoarthritis flare-ups. Keep it around and take one to six grams for a flare-up, or drink one to two cups of cat's claw tea daily to help prevent symptoms.

Curcumin (Osteoarthritis and rheumatoid arthritis): Turmeric is a bright yellow spice used commonly in Indian cooking. It has been known for its medicinal qualities for centuries. The active ingredient of turmeric is called *curcumin*. Curcumin is a very potent antioxidant and has significant anti-inflammatory effects, both of which make it an excellent candidate for relief of arthritis symptoms. Turmeric belongs to the same botanical family as ginger and works against inflammation in much the same way—by blocking the formation of pro-inflammatory eicosanoids. Curcumin's antioxidant power nearly matches that of the OPCs, and it may even boost the effects of the body's natural anti-inflammatory hormone, cortisol. Use a supplement standardized to 90 percent curcumin and take 1,200 mg a day, or 600 mg at breakfast and dinner.

Feverfew (Tanacetum parthenium; rheumatoid arthritis): In Europe, this herb is often used to relieve moderate arthritis symptoms. Feverfew's flavonoids inhibit the production of cyclooxygenase and 5-lipoxygenase enzymes, which means that fewer pro-inflammatory prostaglandins and leukotrienes are created. If you would like to try it, find an extract standardized to 0.2 to 0.4 percent parthenolide and follow the instructions on the container.

Hormones and Rheumatoid Arthritis

Low levels of steroid hormones, such as DHEA, cortisol, and pregnenolone, have been strongly linked to increased risk of rheumatoid arthritis. No matter what type of arthritis you have, you can ask your doctor to measure your body levels of DHEA and cortisol to see whether you're deficient. If you find that you are, replacing them with supplemental hormones may be what you need to bring your body into a more youthful, healthy balance.

DHEA

DHEA (dehydroepiandrosterone) is a steroid hormone made primarily in the adrenal glands that has functions throughout the body. It is the most abundant hormone made by the adrenals. When we are in our twenties, DHEA levels are at their peak. After that, the amount of DHEA steadily declines. By the time we reach our eighties, we have about 10 percent of what we had in our young adult years. The risk of heart disease, diabetes, cancer, weakened immunity, and rheumatoid arthritis increases as levels of DHEA decrease.

Some researchers say that RA may be caused by low DHEA and cortisol levels. Low levels of these hormones lower resistance to certain bacteria that normally exist in the body, allowing them to multiply and cause inflammation in the joints. Replacement of these hormones would, according to this theory, boost immunity and counter inflammation. Cortisol in small, physiologic doses can also have the effect of calming down an overactive and overreactive immune system.

Supplemental DHEA, just enough to restore youthful levels, has many positive effects: it improves memory, immunity, and energy, and brings about a remarkable improvement in well-being—both physical and mental. It has helped in the treatment of osteoporosis and rheumatoid arthritis.

Most of the research into the use of DHEA to treat disease has been done on animals. Although the results of that research have shown this hormone to be a promising therapy for RA, the most compelling evidence in favor of the use of DHEA is the consistency with which very low levels are found in people who have the disease. In one study, levels of DHEA were 86 percent lower in postmenopausal women with RA—and were especially low in the thirty-nine women who were taking synthetic steroid drugs.

DHEA is quite safe for people over forty, in doses equal

to what a youthful body makes. The recommended dose is 5 to 10 mg daily or every other day for women and 10 to 15 mg per day for men. One exception is men with prostate cancer or an abnormal PSA (Prostate Specific Antigen) test, who should not use DHEA. Some women could develop side effects such as the growth of facial hair, male pattern balding, or acne, because DHEA can be converted to the male hormone testosterone. If you are a woman and you experience any masculinizing side effects, cut your dose back to 2 to 5 mg every other day.

Natural Cortisols

Cortisol is a natural anti-inflammatory, and low levels predispose us to fatigue, inability to deal with stress, and inflammation. As you know, when synthetic versions of cortisol—the corticosteroid drugs such as prednisone and prednisolone—are used long-term to counter RA symptoms, the side effects can be devastating.

Endocrinologist William M. Jefferies, M.D., has researched the possible uses and safety of natural cortisols for over thirty years. Natural cortisols are exactly like those made in the body. Rather than giving high doses to suppress inflammation, he advises his patients to use *physiologic* doses—only enough to reverse deficiency and restore hormone balance. In light of research showing cortisol levels to be low in RA patients, the use of natural cortisol makes sense. The case studies he describes in his book, *Safe Uses of Cortisol,* bear this out. People who had been suffering from RA for years gradually improved on 5 to 7.5 mg of hydrocortisone (or Cortef) three to four times a day. If you have often had to use synthetic steroid drugs, you could benefit from natural cortisols. It's much gentler and safer.

Pregnenolone

This steroid hormone is the raw material from which all of the steroid hormones are made. Pregnenolone gives relief from arthritis symptoms to some of those who try it. There was quite a bit of research done on it in the 1940s, which was abandoned when the synthetic corticosteroids came on the market. In the studies, 100 mg two to three times a day was used. You might find it worth a try. It even has the bonus effect of improving memory.

Other Promising Natural Remedies

These following remedies have helped people with both types of arthritis.

Sea Cucumber

Sea vegetables like this one have been used to treat arthritis in China for thousands of years. It isn't really a vegetable at all, but an animal belonging to the same family as sea urchins and starfish. Sea cucumber contains anti-inflammatory compounds that help balance eicosanoids, and also contains chondroitin and sugars called *mucopolysaccharides*—both components of cartilage. Use according to the directions on the container.

Green-Lipped Mussel

In Western Mexico and the South Pacific, extract of green-lipped mussels (*Perna canaliculus*) have been used in the treatment of both rheumatoid arthritis and osteoarthritis for centuries. In clinical trials, the anti-inflammatory compounds they contain have relieved pain, swelling, and stiffness in both types of arthritic disease. Use according to the directions on the container.

Cetyl Myristoleate

In the 1970s, researchers uncovered an interesting characteristic of a specific strain of mice: they didn't get arthritis. They injected them with the same compounds consistently used to induce experimental arthritis in rats, to no avail. When they sought out what in the bodies of these mice might be protective against arthritis, they discovered a fatty acid called cetyl myristoleate (CMO).

CMO had been isolated before, but only in the bodies of sperm whales and beavers. When they isolated it from mice and injected it into rats, it effectively protected the rats from arthritis. Because it proved difficult to rally interest in an unpatentable, natural compound like CMO, the results of these studies sat untouched for years. Recently, CMO has made a comeback, and although no studies on humans have been published in major medical journals, the anecdotal reports of its effectiveness are convincing.

CMO is a fatty acid like the omega-3s and omega-6s, and appears to help eicosanoid balance. It is also thought to have a lubricating effect on joints, which makes it helpful for osteoarthritis that doesn't involve inflammation. The evidence is strong that CMO works best when used along with glucosamine sulfate. If you would like to add it to your arthritis regimen, take about 525 mg per day, or 175 mg three times a day. Take CMO with food.

Coping with Arthritis Pain

We are a culture riddled with aches and pains. Americans take a staggering 30 billion dollars' worth of pain medication a year. Over 100 million suffer from some type of chronic or acute pain; of these, 37 million suffer from arthritis pain, 30 million have frequent headaches, and 15 million cope with cancer pain.

Those who suffer from chronic pain—pain that doesn't go away—often become disabled, depressed, or angry, and their relationships may suffer because of the helplessness they feel. It's no wonder so many turn to over-the-counter and prescription drugs for relief. In this chapter, you'll find out more about some natural, drug-free approaches to dealing with pain.

What Happens When You Hurt

Nerve endings called *nociceptors* are located in the skin and throughout the internal organs, joints, and bones. There can be as many as 1,300 of them in a square inch of skin. For every type of pain, there's a different type of nociceptor. Some pick up on pressure, some on heat, some on inflammation, and some on the sensation of being struck sharply. When tissues are injured by any of the above, the appropriate nociceptors send pain impulses along nerve cell pathways to the brain. Chemicals called *neurotransmitters* help to get the message where it needs to go.

Substance P, a protein present throughout the body, continually stimulates injured nerve endings and keeps pain messages going. When eicosanoids are out of balance, with pro-inflammatory versions predominating, nerve endings are more sensitive and transmit pain messages more quickly.

In the brain, pain impulses travel to a specialized area called the *thalamus.* The thalamus works as a sort of post office, collecting incoming messages and sorting them according to where they need to go next. It sends relevant information on to the *cerebral cortex,* the seat of thought. At this point, we can deal with the pain appropriately: for example, if you are touching a hot pan on the stove, the cerebral cortex evaluates the situation, sees the wisdom of removing your hand from the hot surface, and sends the appropriate signals to the muscles of the arm.

Messages are also sent to the *limbic brain,* the brain's emotional center. This is where our emotional responses to pain come into the picture. Pain is more than a physical sensation. Emotions have a lot to do with where our threshold for pain lies. Our own life experiences and our ability to deal with stress can either diminish or amplify our sensations of pain. If we react to pain with anger, increased tension, or fear, the pain can actually feel worse than if we adopt a more relaxed attitude toward it.

Sensations of pain can also stimulate the *autonomic nervous system,* the part of the nervous system responsible for controlling heartbeat, breathing rate, and blood flow. Stimulation causes pulse and breath rate to rise and directs blood flow away from the organs and into the muscles—the "fight-or-flight" response.

All of this is geared toward letting us know, in no uncertain terms, that something is amiss and needs attention. When we constantly mask pain sensations with drugs, we stifle this important messenger system. On the other hand, if we suffer from pain day in and day out, despite the fact that we have given it all the attention we can muster, we can seek out natural alternatives to ease the discomfort and the stress it can cause. Constant pain can seriously reduce the quality of life and make people difficult to live with. As you've learned—hopefully not firsthand—arthritis pain medications have serious liabilities and should be used only if nothing else does the job.

There are exceptions to this guideline. Pain medication can be a godsend to those on the mend from surgery or injury, who will only need it for a short time. People who are suffering from terminal cancer or other kinds of serious, uncontrollable pain should use all the pain medicines at their disposal. Fear of becoming addicted or experiencing side effects shouldn't keep those who have such serious pain from getting relief. Cancer pain appears to be one of the only conditions for which Americans tend to be *under*medicated.

Managing Arthritis Pain

Physical Therapy

Physical therapy is often prescribed after joint surgery, or to help arthritis patients strengthen weak, painful joints. The physical therapist (PT) will examine you and prescribe specific exercises to help you strengthen and stretch the muscles, tendons, and ligaments around affected joints. You'll be guided through the exercises at first, and once your therapy ends you can continue to do the exercises on your own. The exercises described in chapter 5 are typical of the ones a PT would prescribe to you.

Physical therapy may also include hot and cold packs, whirlpool baths, massage, and TENS (transcutaneous electrical nerve stimulation). In TENS, electrodes are attached in specific places around the painful area. A mild electrical current is passed through the electrodes, and this deadens pain by a mechanism that isn't completely understood. The TENS unit is a small, battery-operated device that you can wear throughout the day once you've been trained in its proper use by a physical therapist.

Occupational Therapy

Occupational therapists help people with physical problems accomplish their day-to-day activities. For someone with severe rheumatoid arthritis in her hands, that might mean fitting special braces to support the joints and teaching her to use writing, cooking, and gardening utensils specially made for arthritic hands. Physical and occupational therapies are covered under most insurance plans.

Acupuncture

In Oriental medicine, it is believed that pain results from energy blockages and stagnation. This energy, called *chi* (chee), can be redistributed and normalized by the insertion of very thin needles at specific points, depending on the location and nature of the pain. Sometimes the needles are only left in for a few minutes, or the acupuncturist may leave them in for an hour. Mild electrical currents may be passed into the needles.

Oriental medicine for pain may also include some other interesting practices, such as:

- *Guasha:* The acupuncturist scrapes the skin with a porcelain spoon.
- *Cupping:* First, the acupuncturist lights an alcohol-soaked gauze pad inside a small glass bottle, creating a vacuum. The gauze is quickly removed, and the bottle is applied to specific areas of the skin.
- *Moxibustion:* Herbs are burned over—not on— painful areas.

Oriental medicine practitioners may also prescribe herbs to their patients that bring blood flow to where the pain is and direct the body's innate healing energy to those places that need it.

Clinical studies have shown acupuncture and other Oriental medicine practices to be effective at relieving pain when done by a skilled practitioner. There's more evidence in favor of its use in osteoarthritis, but there are other studies that support its use against rheumatoid arthritis pain. In two Chinese studies, researchers found that acupuncture toned down the out-of-control immune responses typical of RA.

To find an acupuncturist in your part of the world, call the American Association of Oriental Medicine at (610) 266-1433. You can also check your local yellow pages for licensed acupuncturists, who will have L.Ac. after their names.

Feldenkrais and Alexander Work: Movement Re-Education

Over our lifetimes, we develop unhealthy movement patterns and ways of carrying ourselves. Sitting hunched over a desk and over the wheel of a car for years and years can result in a chronically hunched posture, which is carried through all the body's movements. A shoulder injury can cause poor alignment even years after it has healed, because of habitual tensing of the muscles in an unconscious attempt to protect the shoulder from further damage. When the spine is out of alignment, it affects joints in the shoulders, hips, knees, ankles, and feet. Pain is often the result of the chronic muscle tension necessary to hold the body in unnatural alignment. These patterns may feel right to us, but only because they are habitual.

The teachings of Moshe Feldenkrais and F. M. Alexander address these issues. Therapists trained in these teachings will help you re-learn the most basic movements, many that you may never have given any conscious thought to: sitting in a chair, climbing a staircase, walking, going from sitting to lying down.

How does movement re-education relieve arthritis pain? When we don't pay attention to how we sit, stand, walk, and lie down, we adopt movement patterns and postures that put uneven stresses on the joints. These patterns don't change quickly, and it may take a few months before you experience real pain relief. But if your arthritis pain is being aggravated by the tensions in your present movement patterns, it's worth it to invest some time and energy in going to the root of those problems.

An Alexander teacher uses gentle contact with the

hands to re-educate the body, while it is both still and in motion. The student has to pay close attention and participate. It's a wonderful, gentle way to get back in touch with your body and to learn to use it in the way it was designed to be used.

Feldenkrais, too, seeks to re-educate the body through a series of very simple exercises that feel good and increase awareness. You can find a Feldenkrais practitioner by calling the Feldenkrais Guild of North America at (800) 775-2118. There isn't any national organization you can contact to find an Alexander teacher; you may need to check your phone book or ask around.

Therapeutic Massage

The manipulation of soft tissues by a trained massage therapist has many benefits. It improves circulation and releases knotted muscles. A skilled practitioner can focus on painful areas, encouraging the body to heal those places. Massage's pain-relieving effects are probably largely due to how relaxing it is (if it isn't, you're seeing the wrong massage therapist). It increases levels of *serotonin,* a "feel-good" neurotransmitter, and decreases levels of stress hormones.

There are many different kinds of massage. The best types for RA patients are very gentle. Don't let a massage therapist deeply massage or otherwise manipulate inflamed joints. The best way to work on those areas is by doing your range of motion exercises.

Those with osteoarthritis can try more vigorous forms of massage, including deep tissue work, acupressure (where the therapist applies pressure to specific points), shiatsu (a Japanese form of massage that incorporates acupressure and manipulation of the joints to open up energy channels), and sports massage. Communicate closely with your massage therapist. Tell her about your arthritis symptoms in detail and don't be afraid to ask her to back off if she's causing you a lot of discomfort.

More and more insurers are covering massage therapy when it's warranted for pain. Physical therapists sometimes do massage as part of the treatments they deliver. Check with your insurance company to see whether it's covered on your plan.

To find a licensed massage therapist in your area, call the American Massage Therapy Association at (847) 864-0123 or check your yellow pages for licensed massage therapists (LMTs). Ask family or friends whether they can recommend anyone to you.

Emotional Work and Counseling

Emotions have a lot to do with our experience of pain. This helps to explain why two people's arthritic joints, which look the same on an X-ray, may cause little or no pain in one person and debilitating pain in the other. If you are constantly wound up, stressed, and unhappy, your body's natural "feel-good" chemicals, the *endorphins,* are suppressed, and you feel pain more acutely.

Work with some type of counselor—whether it's a psychologist, clinical social worker, or a spiritual counselor such as a minister or rabbi—to examine any emotional, spiritual, or interpersonal issues that are causing you stress. Qualified counselors help you to keep things in perspective and give you valuable tools for coping with adversity. Once you start doing this kind of work with a counselor, you'll become more relaxed.

If all else fails, go out and rent your favorite funny movie and laugh. Laughter is an excellent stimulator of endorphin release.

Hypnosis

In a session of hypnosis, the hypnotist helps the patient reach a state of deep relaxation. While the patient is "under," the hypnotist gives verbal suggestions for changing perceptions and experiences of pain. There is plentiful clinical evidence of its effectiveness. Hypnotherapy for pain actually changes levels of biochemicals in the body that cause or intensify painful sensations.

To find a hypnotherapist, call the American Institute of Hypnotherapy at (800) 634-9766, or check your yellow pages for licensed clinical hypnotherapists.

Yoga Therapy

Yoga therapists are specially trained to teach yoga as a healing art. They learn what poses are beneficial in various conditions and teach their clients how to gain those benefits. Yoga therapy lengthens and relaxes the muscles, works the joints through their full ranges of motion, and improves circulation. The therapist may also teach breathing exercises to help you control "fight-or-flight" responses to pain. Contact your local yoga studios to find out whether they have any yoga therapists on staff.

Guided Imagery

In a session of guided imagery, a specially trained therapist will talk you through some imaginary scenarios designed to help ease pain or relieve stress. If you have pain in your knee, for example, the therapist might help you imagine a gentle, healing hand massaging the joint. Once you've done the exercises with a therapist, you should be able to do them on your own at home.

If you would like to try guided imagery on your own at

home, you can purchase relaxation tapes to listen to, or imagine yourself in your absolutely favorite place. For example, you could picture a tropical beach, adding all the details: warm breeze, warm sand, the sound of the waves and wafting palm fronds, the blue of the ocean, the calls of the sea birds, and the smell of the flowers.

Helping Yourself Through Pain

Here are some tools you can use to self-treat pain.

Moist Heat: A long, hot shower or bath can do wonders for relieving pain. In the shower, aim the shower head at the places that hurt. If you have access to a Jacuzzi, relax in the tub and point the jets toward sore areas. Aromatic oils in the water can help you relax tight muscles; try myrrh oil (which is a natural pain reliever) or lavender oil.

Relaxation techniques: When in pain, people tend to tense their muscles around the painful area. For example, if you have arthritis in your right shoulder, the muscles all around your shoulder joint, upper neck, and back will tense up. This is an unconscious way of "guarding" that area, to try to lessen the discomfort and prevent further injury. As a result of all this excess tension, other parts of the body fall out of balance and more tensions and tightnesses result. In the end, it can throw an already out-of-balance body even further out of whack, amplifying feelings of pain.

Relaxation techniques loosen muscles and joints. Here's a handy method for getting to a state of deep relaxation:

1. Lie on your back in a comfortable position, eyes closed. You may want to turn on some soft, meditative music.

2. Send your attention all the way down to your toes. Tense the muscles in your toes for two to four deep breaths, and then relax them. Then, send your attention to the soles of your feet, and tense and release them. Do the same with your ankles, your calves, the front of your shins, your knees, thighs, your buttocks, your belly, fingers, arms, chest, shoulders, neck, face, and scalp.
3. Lie still for a few minutes, enjoying your feeling of total relaxation.

Guided imagery and meditation are other good methods for becoming relaxed.

Meditation: In chapter 5, you learned a meditation exercise. Meditation is an excellent way to bring yourself "into the present" and into whatever sensations are going on in your body. We spend so much energy thinking about what has already happened or what will happen, that we rarely make time to simply relax and be in this very moment.

This is especially true of people who are often in pain. The natural instinct in the face of pain is to try to escape it, to tune out and preoccupy ourselves. Much of the discomfort people in pain end up experiencing springs from their desperation to escape it. When we learn to meditate, we learn to look directly at what we are experiencing— and in most cases, it isn't really as bad as we thought. A study by John Kabat-Zinn, Ph.D., included fifty-one chronic pain patients who hadn't responded to medical treatment. After a ten-week stress reduction and relaxation program, which included a meditation practice called "mindfulness meditation," 65 percent of the patients showed significant improvement. In another study, people who regularly practiced transcendental meditation had much milder stress responses to pain than those without meditation training.

There are many excellent teachers of meditation all over the world, so do find one that suits you and works well for you.

Magnet Therapy: This entails the use of specially designed magnets for the reduction of pain. Available in many shapes and sizes, these magnets are applied in a specific pattern around painful areas. No one is sure exactly how magnet therapy works, but it appears to offer some relief to many who use them. In some, magnets increase pain sensations at first but eventually offer total relief. Many people who use them swear by them. They can be worn for several hours at a time, but must be removed for a while each day.

Some say that magnets work by improving circulation in painful areas, flushing inflammatory and pain-stimulating biochemicals out and bringing fresh blood and nutrients in. Others guess that the magnets alter the contraction of muscle cells, or may block the passage of pain messages to the brain.

Magnets only work as long as you wear them. They don't offer any long-term curative effects. If you are interested in using magnets for pain, call the North American Academy for Magnetic Therapy at (800) 457-1853 to find out more. People who wear pacemakers, are pregnant, or have bleeding disorders should not use magnets.

Herbs and Other Natural Remedies for Pain and Anxiety

You'll probably want to keep some or all of these remedies in your herbal medicine cabinet. Some are especially effective at soothing pain, while others are good for relaxation of tense muscles and for improving sleep quality.

Capsaicin: Cayenne pepper contains *capsaicin,* a chemical known to have healing properties against many chronic diseases—including heart disease and cancer. Capsaicin can also be found in many commercially available topical pain relievers. It deadens pain by depleting the nerves of substance P, the biochemical that transmits pain messages from the joints to the brain. If the pain messages don't travel to the brain, the pain isn't felt.

Hundreds of studies support the use of capsaicin creams for temporary pain relief. It must be applied daily for continued relief, and in some people it may take a few weeks to get results. Use a cream that contains 0.025 percent capsaicin—you should be able to find one on your drugstore's shelves. Be careful not to get any residue in your eyes or mouth, because it will burn delicate mucous membranes. Wash your hands carefully right after use.

White Willow Bark (Salicix cortex): Salicylate drugs (primarily aspirin) were first derived from white willow bark. This herb is a milder, natural version of aspirin. A standardized extract containing 60 to 100 mg salicin per dose may help relieve mild osteoarthritis pain.

Kava kava: Derived from a South Pacific pepper plant, kava has traditionally been made into a ceremonial drink in the South Pacific islands. The beverage made from kava root brings about contentment, relaxation, and increased sociability in those who consume it—much like alcohol does, but without the damage to the liver or loss of faculties caused by alcohol. Kava is most commonly used in the Western world as an anti-anxiety supplement.

Kava is quite safe and effective against anxiety and depression caused by chronic pain. It even appears to have pain-killing properties. You can take it during the day in small doses, and you can take larger doses at night if you have trouble sleeping. Look for an extract containing 70 percent kavalactones, and take 100 mg three times daily for anxiety and pain relief, or take 300 mg right before bed to help you sleep.

DL-phenylalanine (DLPA): L-Phenylalanine is an essential amino acid that is important for alertness, memory, and mood. D-Phenylalanine is also an amino acid, with a special quality: it raises levels of endorphins. Remember, endorphins are natural painkillers made in the brain.) When combined to form DLPA, the two have potent pain-relieving effects, especially against arthritis and back pain.

DLPA is transformed into the neurotransmitters dopamine, noradrenaline, and adrenaline, and these neurotransmitters are important regulators of mood, energy, and general well-being. To relieve chronic pain or depression, take 1,000 to 2,000 mg a day at first. If this isn't enough, you can take up to 3,000 mg a day. If you have high blood pressure, be sure to monitor it while using DLPA—it can cause it to rise. Only use DLPA for short-term relief (three weeks or less at a time). Long-term use can interfere with the body's balance of amino acids and can pose danger to liver and kidneys.

Valerian: This herb is a wonderfully gentle sleep aid and muscle relaxant. Herbalists have used it for centuries to relieve anxiety, panic attacks, and nervous tension. You can use it to help you sleep more deeply at night, or to relax tight, cramped muscles during the day. Don't exceed the recommended dose on the container, because high doses can cause paralysis and weakened heartbeat. Valerian can make some people weepy.

Melatonin: Melatonin is a hormone made in the pineal gland, a tiny organ nestled in the brain. It is the hormone that tells the body when it's time to go to sleep. When darkness falls, melatonin is pumped into the bloodstream, and we become sleepy.

The prevalence of electric lighting has our pineal glands quite confused. As long as rooms are brightly lit, melatonin secretion stays low. Aging also decreases our melatonin secretion. When melatonin is low, sleep quality is compromised. When you're dealing with pain, it can be hard enough to sleep as it is, and anyone who has ever laid awake at night in pain knows how awful it can be. The next day, you're irritable and tense, and your pain is made worse by your lack of sleep.

When it seems too hard to sleep through the night, use melatonin to help you fall asleep and stay asleep. A 1 mg sublingual tablet is all you'll need. Slip it beneath your tongue a half hour before going to bed.

References

CHAPTER TWO

Bland, J. H., and S. M. Cooper. "Osteoarthritis: a review of
the cell biology involved and evidence for reversibility.
Management rationally related to known genesis and
pathophysiology," *Seminars in Arthritis and Rheumatism*
1984;14:106–33.

CHAPTER THREE

Bennett, W. M. "Drug-related renal dysfunction in the
elderly." *Geriatric Nephrology and Urology,* 1999;9(1):
21–5.

Bjarnsason, I. "Forthcoming NSAIDs: are they really de-
void of side effects?" *Italian Journal of Gastroenterology
and Hepatology* 1999;31Suppl:927–36.

Bland, J. H., and S. M. Cooper. "Osteoarthritis: a review of
the cell biology involved and evidence for reversibility.
Management rationally related to known genesis and

pathophysiology" *Seminars in Arthritis and Rheumatism* 1984;14:106–33.

Brooks, P. M., and S. R. Potter. "NSAID and arthritis—help or hindrance?" *Journal of Rheumatology* 1982;9: 3–5.

Fung, H. B., and H. L. Kirschenbaum. "Selective cyclooxygenase-2 inhibitors for therapy of arthritis." *Clinical Therapeutics* July 1999;21(7): 1131–57.

Kaplan-Machlis, B., et al. "The cyclooxygenase-2 inhibitors: safety and effectiveness," *Annals of Pharmacotherapy* 1999 September;33(9):979–88.

LaCorte, R., et al. "Prophylaxis and therapy of NSAID-induced gastrointestinal disorders." *Drug Safety* June 1999;20(6):527–43.

McKenna, F. "COX-2: separating myth from reality." *Scandinavian Journal of Rheumatology Supplement,* 1999; 109:19–29.

Mindell, E., and V. Hopkins. *Prescription Alternatives,* Second Edition. Los Angeles: Keats Publishing, 1999.

Murphy, P. J., B. L. Myers, and P. Badia. "Nonsteroidal anti-inflammatory drugs alter body temperature and suppress melatonin in humans." *Physiology and Behavior* January 1996;59(1):133–9.

Newman, N. M., and R. S. M. Ling. "Acetabular bond destruction related to non-steroidal anti-inflammatory drugs," *Lancet,* 1985; ii:11–13

Pelletier, J. P. "The influence of tissue cross-talking on osteoarthritis progression: role of nonsteroidal anti-inflammatory drugs." *Osteoarthritis and Cartilage* July 1999;7(4):374–6.

Perry, G. H., M. J. D. Smith, and C. G. Whiteside, "Spontaneous recovery of the hip joint space in degenerative hip disease." *Annals of Rheumatic Diseases* 1972; 31:440–8.)

Peskar, B. M., et al. "Role of prostaglandins in gastroprotection." *Digestive Disease Science* September 1998;43(9 Suppl):23S–29S.

Sears, B., and B. Lawren. *Enter The Zone.* New York: Regan Books, an imprint of HarperCollins Publishers, 1995.

Shanna, S., A. Prasad, and K. S. Anand. "Nonsteroidal anti-inflammatory drugs in the management of pain and inflammation: a basis for drug selection." *American Journal of Therapeutics* January 1, 1999;6(1):3–11.

Solomon, L. "Drug-induced arthropathy and necrosis of the femoral head." *Journal of Bone and Joint Surgery* 1973;55B:246–51.

Vassilopoulos, D., C. Camisa, and R. M. Strauss, "Selected drug complications and treatment conflicts in the presence of coexistent diseases." *Rheumatic Disease Clinics of North America* August 1999;25(3):745–777.

Weatherby C., and L. Gordin. *The Arthritis Bible.* Rochester, VT: Healing Arts Press, 1999.

CHAPTER FOUR

Bland, J. *Intestinal Toxicity and Inner Cleansing.* New Canaan, CT: Keats Publishing, 1991.

Chou, C. T., J. Uksila, and P. Toivanen. "Enterobacterial antibodies in Chinese patients with rheumatoid arthritis and ankylosing spondylitis." *Clinical and Experimental Rheumatology* March–April 1998;16(2):161–4.

DeKeyser, F., et al. "Bowel inflammation and the spondyloarthropathies." *Rheumatic Disease Clinics of North America* November 1998;24(4):785–813, ix–x.

Feldman, M., et al. "Effects of aging and gastritis on gastric acid and pepsin secretion in humans: a prospective study." *Gastroenterology* April 1996;110(4):1043–52.

Fuhrman, J. *Fasting—and Eating—for Health.* St. Martin's Griffin, New York, 1998.

Galland, L. "Nutrition and candidiasis." *Journal of Orthomolecular Psychiatry* 1985;15:50–60.

Glick, L. "Deglycrrhizinated liquorice in peptic ulcer." *Lancet.* 1982;ii:817.

Golan, R. *Optimal Wellness.* New York: Ballantine Books, 1995.

Goodrick, C. L., et al. "Effects of intermittent feeding upon growth, activity and lifespan in rats allowed voluntary exercise." *Experimental Aging Research* 1983;9:1477–94.

Guslandi, M., A. Pellegrini, and M. Sorghi. "Gastric mucosal defences in the elderly." *Gerontology* July 1999;45(4):206–208.

Guslandi, M., and E. Ballarin. "Assessment of the 'mucus-bicarbonate' barrier in the stomach of patients with chronic gastric disorders." *Clinica Chimica Acta* December 29, 1984;144(2–3):133–6.

Hafstrom, I., et al. "Effects of fasting on disease activity, neutrophil function, fatty acid composition, and leukotriene biosynthesis in patients with rheumatoid arthritis." *Arthritis and Rheumatism* 1988;31:585.

Hojgaard, L., A. Mertz-Nielsen, and S. J. Rune. "Peptic ulcer pathophysiology: acid, bicarbonate, and mucosal function." *Scandinavian Journal of Gastroenterology* 1996 Suppl;216:10–15.

Kenyon, J. N. "Food sensitivity, a search for underlying causes: case study of 12 patients," *Acupuncture and Electrotherapy Research* 1986;11(1):1–13.

Kroker, G. F., et al. "Fasting and rheumatoid arthritis: A multicenter study." *Clinical Ecology* 1984;2(3):137–144.

Masoro, E. J., I. Shimokawa, and B. P. Yu. "Retardation of the aging process in rats by food restriction." *Annals of the New York Academy of Science* 1990;337–52.

McColl, K. E. L., et al. "Eradication of Helicobacter pylori in functional dyspepsia." *British Journal of Medicine* 1999;319:451.

Murray, M., and J. Pizzorno. *Encyclopedia of Natural Medicine.* Rocklin, CA: Prima Publishing, 1991.

Panush, R. S. "Delayed reactions to foods: food allergy and rheumatic disease." *Annals of Allergy* 1986;56:500–503.

Sartor, R. B. "Review article: Role of the enteric microflora in the pathogenesis of intestinal inflammation and arthritis." *Aliementary Pharmacology and Therapy* December 1997;11 Suppl3:17–22.

Shiratori, K., S. Watanabe, and T. Takeuchi. "Effect of licorice extract (Fm100) on release of secretin and exocrine pancreatic secretion in humans." *Pancreas* 1986;1(6):483–7.

Silveri, F., et al. "Serum levels of insulin in overweight patients with osteoarthritis of the knee." *Journal of Rheumatology* October 1994;21(10):1899–902.

Tewari, S. N., and A. K. Wilson. "Deglycrrhizinated liquorice in duodenal ulcer." *Practitioner* 1972;210: 820–5.

Truss, C. O. "The role of Candida albicans in human illness." *Journal of Orthomolecular Psychiatry* 1981;10: 228–238.

Wilson, D. E. "The role of prostaglandins in gastric mucosal protection." *Trans Am Clin Climatol Assoc* 1995; 107:99–113.

Yashiro, N. "Clinico-psychological and pathophysiological studies on fasting therapy." *Sapporo Medical Journal* 1986;55(2):125–136.

CHAPTER FIVE

Adderly, B. *The Arthritis Cure Fitness Solution.* Washington, D.C.: Regnery Publishing, 1999.

Bostrom, C., et al. "Effect of static and dynamic shoulder rotator exercises in women with rheumatoid arthritis: a randomised comparison of impairment, disability, handicap, and health." *Scandinavian Journal of Rheumatology* 1998;27(4):281–90.

Buckwalter, J. A. "Osteoarthritis and articular cartilage use, disuse, and abuse: experimental studies," *Journal of Rheumatology.* February 1995 Suppl;43:13–5.

Cooper, K. *Arthritis: Your Complete Exercise Guide.* Champaign, IL: Cooper Clinic and Research Institute Fitness Series, Human Kinetics Publishing, 1992.

Cohen, D. *Arthritis: Stop Suffering, Start Moving.* New York: Walter and Company, 1995.

Ellert, G., RN, BSN, and B. Koehler. *The Arthritis Exercise Book: Gentle Joint by Joint Exercise to Keep You Flexible and Independent.* Lincolnwood, IL: NTC/Contemporary Publishers, 1990.

Hurley, M. V. "The role of muscle weakness in the pathogenesis of osteoarthritis." *Rheumatic Disease Clinics of North America* May 1999;25(2):vi, 283–98.

Minor, M. A. "Exercise in the therapy of osteoarthritis." *Rheumatic Disease Clinics of North America* May 1999; 25(2):viii, 397–415.

Sobel, D., A. C. Klein, and J. Bland. *Arthritis: What Exercises Work.* New York: St. Martin's Press, 1995.

Van den Ende, C. H., et al. "Dynamic exercise therapy in rheumatoid arthritis—a systematic review." *British Journal of Rheumatology* January 1998;37(6):677–87.

CHAPTER SIX

Aaseth, J., M. Haugen, and O. Forre. "Rheumatoid arthritis and metal compounds—perspectives on the role of oxygen radical detoxification." *Analyst* January 1998; 123(1):3–6.

Bang, B., et al. "Reduced 25-hydroxyvitamin D levels in primary Sjogren's syndrome. Correlations to disease manifestations." *Scandinavian Journal of Rheumatology* 1999;28(3):180–3.

Bates, C. J. "Proline and hydroxyline excretion and vitamin C status in elderly human subjects." *Clinical Science and Molecular Medicine* 1977;52:525–43.

Calder, P. C. "n-3 polyunsaturated fatty acids and cytokine production in health and disease." *Annals of Nutrition and Metabolism* 1997;41(4):203–34.

Cichoke, A. J. "Treating rheumatoid arthritis with enzymes." *Townsend Letter for Doctors and Patients.* January 1996;32–34.

Cohen, A., and J. Goldman. "Bromelain therapy in rheumatoid arthritis." *Pennsylvania Medical Journal* 1964;67:27–30.

Comstock, G. W., et al. "Serum concentrations of alpha tocopherol, beta-carotene, and retinol preceding the diagnosis of rheumatoid arthritis and systemic lupus erythematosus." *Annals of Rheumatic Diseases* 1997;56: 323–5.

Das, U. N. "Beneficial effect of eicosapentaenoic and docosahexaenoic acids in the management of systemic lupus erythematosus and its relationship to the cytokine network." *Prostaglandins, Leukotrienes, and Essential Fatty Acids* September 1994;51(3):207–13.

DeMarco, D. M., D. Santoli, and R. B. Zurier. "Effects of fatty acids on proliferation and activation of human synovial compartment lymphocytes." *Journal of Leukocyte Biology* November 1994;56(5):612–5.

Edmonds, S. E., et al. "Putative analgesic activity of repeated oral doses of vitamin E in the treatment of rheumatoid arthritis. Results of a prospective placebo controlled double blind trial." *Annals of Rheumatic Disease* November 1997;56(11):649–55.

Fawzy, A. A., B. S. Vishwanath, and R. C. Franson. "Inhibition of human non-pancreatic phospholipases A2 by retinoids and flavonoids. Mechanism of action." *Agents and Actions* December 1988;25(3–4):394–400.

Gabor, M., et al. "Effects of benzopyrone derivatives on simultaneously induced croton oil ear oedema and carageenan paw oedema in rats." *Acta Physiologica Hungaria* 1985;65(2):235–40.

Geusens, P., et al. "Long term effect of omega-3 fatty acid supplementation in active rheumatoid arthritis: a 12-month, double-blind controlled study." *Arthritis and Rheumatism* 1994;37(6):824–29.

Hansen, T. M., et al. "Treatment of rheumatoid arthritis with prostaglandin E1 precursors cis-linoleic acid and gamma-linoleic acid." *Scandinavian Journal of Rheumatology* 1983;12:85–8.

Heller, A., et al. "Lipid mediators in inflammatory disorders," *Drugs,* April 1998;55(4):487–96.

Horrobin, D. F., et al. "The regulation of prostaglandin E1 formation: a candidate for one of the fundamental mechanisms involved in the action of vitamin C." *Medical Hypotheses* 1979;5(8):849–858.

Jacob, Stanley W., Ronald M. Lawrence, and Martin Zucker. *The Miracle of MSM: The Natural Solution for Pain,* New York: G. P. Putnam's Sons, 1999.

Jonas, W. B., C. P. Rapoza, and W. F. Blair. "The effect of

niacinimide on osteoarthritis: a pilot study." *Inflammation Research* 1996;45:330–4; also, A. Hoffer, "Treatment of arthritis by nicotinic acid and nicotinamide," *Canadian Medican Association Journal* 1959;81:235–39.

Jones, G., et al. "Allelic variation in the vitamin D receptor, lifestyle factors and lumbar spinal degenerative disease." *Annals of Rheumatic Disease* February 1998;57(2):94–9.

Kheir-Eldin, A. A., et al. "Biochemical changes in arthritic rats under the influence of vitamin E," *Agents and Actions,* July 1992;36(3–4):300–5.

Kjeldsen-Kragh, J., et al. "Dietary omega-3 fatty acid supplementation and naproxen treatment in patients with rheumatoid arthritis." *Journal of Rheumatology* October 1992;19(10):1531–6.

Kose, K., et al. "Plasma selenium levels in rheumatoid arthritis," *Biological Trace Element Research,* Summer 1996;53(1–3):51–6.

Kremer, J. M., et al. "Effects of high-dose fish oil on rheumatoid arthritis after stopping NSAIDs: Clinical and immune correlates." *Arthritis and Rheumatism* 1995;38(8):1107–14.

Krystal, G., et al. "Stimulation of DNA synthesis by ascorbate in cultures of articular chondrocytes," *Arthritis and Rheumatism,* 1982;25:525–43.

Kumakura, S., M. Yamashita, and S. Tsurufuji. "Effect of bromelain on kaolin-induced inflammation in rats," *European Journal of Pharmacology* June 10, 1988;150(3): 295–301.

Lane, N. E., et al. "Serum vitamin D levels and incident changes of radiographic hip osteoarthritis: a longitudinal study. Study of Osteoporosis Fractures Research Group." *Arthritis and Rheumatism* May 1999;42(5):854–60.

Larsson, P., et al. "A vitamin D analogue (MC 1288) has immunomodulatory properties and suppresses collagen-induced arthritis (CIA) without causing hypercalcemia." *Clinics in Experimental Immunology* November 1998;114(2):277–83.

Lau, C. S., K. D. Morley, and J. J. Belch. "Effects of fish oil supplementation on non-steroidal anti-inflammatory drug requirement in patients with mild rheumatoid arthritis—a double-blind placebo controlled study." *British Journal of Rheumatology* November 1993;32(11): 982–9.

Machtey, I., and L. Ouaknine , "Tocopherol in osteoarthritis: a controlled pilot study." *Journal of the American Geriatric Society* 1978;25(7):328.

Mahmud, Z., and S. M. Ali, "Role of vitamin A and E in spondylosis." *Bangladesh Medical Research Council Bulletin* April 1992;18(1):47–59.

Mantizioris, E., et al. "Dietary substitution with alpha-linoleic acid-rich vegetable oil increases eicosapentaenoic acid concentrations in tissues." *American Journal of Clinical Nutrition* 1994;59:1304–1309.

Masson, M. "Bromelain in the treatment of blunt injuries to the musculoskeletal system. A case observation study by an orthopedic surgeon in private practice." *Fortschritte der Medezin* 1995;113(9):303–06.

McAlindon, T. E., et al. "Do antioxidant micronutrients protect against the development of knee osteoarthritis?" *Arthritis and Rheumatism* 1996;39:648–56.

———. "Relation of dietary intake and serum levels of vitamin D to progression of osteoarthritis of the knee among participants in the Framingham study." *Annals of Internal Medicine* 1996;125:353–9.

"Monograph: Bromelain," *Alternative Medicine Review,* August 1998;3(4):302–5.

Moreno-Reyes, R., et al. "Kashin-Beck osteoarthropathy in rural Tibet in relation to selenium and iodine status." *New England Journal of Medicine* October 15, 1998; 339(16):1112–20.

Nordstrom, D. C., et al. "Alpha-linoleic acid in the treatment of rheumatoid arthritis. A double-blind, placebo-controlled and randomized study: flaxseed vs. safflower seed." *Rheumatology International* 1995;14(6):231–34.

Oelzner, P., et al. "Relationship between diseased activity and serum levels of vitamin D metabolites and PTH in rheumatoid arthritis." *Calcified Tissue International* March 1998;62(3):193–8.

Oxholm, P., et al. "Essential fatty acid status in cell membranes and plasma of patients with primary Sjogren's syndrome. Correlations to clinical and immunologic variables using a new model for classification and assessment of disease manifestations." *Prostaglandins, Leukotrienes, and Essential Fatty Acids* October 1998;59(4):239–45.

Rao, C. N., V. H. Rao, and B. Steinmann. "Bioflavonoid-mediated stabilization of collagen in adjuvant-induced arthritis." *Scandinavian Journal of Rheumatology* 1983; 12(1):39–42.

————. "Influence of bioflavonoids on the collagen metabolism in rats with adjuvant induced arthritis." *Italian Journal of Biochemistry* January–February 1981; 30(1):54–62.

Sakai, A., et al. "Large-dose ascorbic acid administration suppresses the development of arthritis in adjuvant-infected rats." *Archives of Orthopedic Trauma Surgery* 1999;119(3–4):121–6.

Sangha, O., and G. Stucki. "Vitamin E in therapy of rheumatic diseases." *Zeitchrift fur Rheumatologie* August 1998;57(4):207–14.

Sasaki, S., et al. "Low-selenium diet, bone, and articular cartilage in rats." *Nutrition* November–December 1994;10(6):538–43.

Saso, L., et al. "Inhibition of protein denaturation by fatty acids, bile salts, and other natural substances: a new hypothesis for the mechanism of action of fish oil in rheumatic diseases." *Japanese Journal of Pharmacology* January 1999;79(1):89–99.

Sato, M., et al. "Quercetin, a bioflavonoid, inhibits the induction of interleukin 8 and monocyte chemoattractant protein-1 expression by tumor necrosis factor-alpha in cultured human synovial cells." *Journal of Rheumatology* September 1997;24(9):1680–4.

Simopoulos, A. P. "Omega-3 fatty acids in health and disease and in growth and development." *American Journal of Clinical Nutrition* September 1991;54(3):438–63.

Steffen, C., et al. "Enzyme therapy in comparison with immune complex determinations in chronic polyarthritis." *Zeitschrift fur Rheumatologie* March–April 1985;44(2):51–6.

Steffen, C., and J. Menzel. "Enzyme breakdown of immune complexes." *Zeitschrift Rheumatologie* September–October 1983;42(5):249–55.

———. "Basic studies on enzyme therapy of immune complex diseases." *Wiener Klinische Wochenschrift* April 1985;12;97(8):376–85

Stone, J., et al. "Inadequate calcium, folic acid, vitamin E, zinc, and selenium intake in rheumatoid arthritis patients: results of a dietary survey." *Arthritis and Rheumatism* December 1997;27(3):180–5.

Taussig, S. "The mechanism of the physiological action of bromelain," *Medical Hypotheses,* 1980;6:99–104.

Tetlow, L. C., et al. "Vitamin D receptors in the rheumatoid lesion: expression by chondrocytes, macrophages, and synoviocytes." *Annals of Rheumatic Diseases* February 1999;58(2):118–21.

Tixier, J. M., et al. "Evidence by in vivo and in vitro studies that binding of pycnogenols to elastin effects its rate of degradation by elastases." *Biochemical Pharmacology* 1884;33(24):3933–39.

Tuncer, S., et al. "Trace element and magnesium levels and superoxide dismutase activity in rheumatoid arthritis." *Biological Trace Element Research* May 1999;68(2):137–42.

Vassilopoulos, D., et al. "Gammalinolenic acid and dihomogammalinolenic acid suppress the CD-3 mediated signal transduction pathway in human T cells." *Clinical Immunology and Immunopathology* June 1997;83(3):237–44.

Vellini, M., et al. "Possible involvement of eicosanoids in the pharmacological action of bromelain." *Arzneimittelforschung* 1986;36(1):110–12.

Virgili, F., H. Kobuchi, and L. Packer, "Procyanidins extracted from Pinus maritima (Pycnogenol): scavengers of free radical species and modulators of nitrogen monoxide metabolism in activated murine RAW 264.7 macrophages." *Free Radical Biology and Medicine* May 1998;24(7–8):1120–9.

Walker, J. A., et al. "Attenuation of contraction-induced skeletal muscle injury by bromelain." *Medicine and Science in Sports and Exercise* January 1992;24(1):20–5.

Weatherby, Craig, and Leonid Gordin. Rochester, VT: *The Arthritis Bible,* Healing Arts Press, 1999.

Zurier, R. B., et al. "Gamma-linoleic acid treatment of rheumatoid arthritis." *Arthritis and Rheumatism* 1996; 39:1808–17.

CHAPTER SEVEN

Ammon, H. P., et al. "Mechanism of anti-inflammatory actions of curcumin and boswellic acids." *Journal of Ethnopharmacology* March 1993;38(2–3):113–9.

Austin, S. "The Confusion Over Chondroitin." *Quarterly Review of Natural Medicine* Summer 1997:125–126.

———. "Double-blinded evidence supports cetyl myristoleate." *Quarterly Review of Natural Medicine* Winter 1997;315–316.

Barclay, T. S., C. Tsourounis, and G. M. McCart. "Glucosamine," *Annals of Pharmacotherapy* May 1998;32(5):574–9.

Bassleer, C., L. Rovati, and P. Franchimont. "Stimulation of proteoglycan production by glucosamine sulfate in chondrocytes isolated from human osteoarthritic articular cartilage in vitro." *Osteoarthritis and Cartilage* November 1998;6(6):427–34.

Caughey, D. E., et al. "Perna canaliculus in the treatment of rheumatoid arthritis." *European Journal of Rheumatology and Inflammation* 1983;6(2):197–200.

Cranton, E., and W. Fryer. *Resetting the Clock,* M. Evans and Company, New York, NY, 1996.

DaCamara, C. C., and G. V. Dowless. "Glucosamine sulfate for osteoarthritis." *Annals of Pharmacotherapy* May 1998;32(5):580–7.

Deal, C. L., and R. W. Moskowitz. "Nutraceuticals as therapeutic agents in osteoarthritis. The role of glucosamine, chondroitin sulfate, and collagen hydrolysate." *Rheumatic Diseases Clinics of North America* May 1999;25(2):379–95.

Diehl, W., and E. L. May. "Cetyl myristoleate isolated from Swiss albino mice: an apparent protective agent against adjuvant arthritis in rats." *Journal of Pharmaceutical Science* March 1994;83(3):296–9.

Jefferies, W. M. "The etiology of rheumatoid arthritis." *Medical Hypotheses* August 1998;51(2):111–4.

———. *Safe Uses of Cortisol.* Springfield, IL: Charles C. Thomas, Publisher, 1996.

Jobin, C., et al. "Curcumin blocks cytokine-mediated NF-kappaB activation and proinflammatory gene expression by inhibiting inhibitory factor 1-kappaB kinase activity." *Journal of Immunology* September 15, 1999;163(6):3474–3483.

Keplinger, K., et al. "Unicaria tomentosa (Wiild) DC—ethnomedicinal use and new pharmacological, toxicological and botanical results." *Journal of Ethnopharmacology* January 1999;64(1):23–34.

Leffler, C. T., et al. "Glucosamine, chondroitin, and manganese ascorbate for degenerative joint disease of the knee or low back: a randomized, double-blind, placebo-controlled pilot study." *Milano Medicine* February 1999;164(2):85–91.

Masi, A. T., R. T. Chatterton, and J. C. Aldag. "Perturbations of hypothalamic-pituitary-gonadal axis and adrenal androgen functions in rheumatoid arthritis: an odyssey of hormonal relationships to the disease." *Annals of the New York Academy of Sciences* June 22, 1999;876:53–62; discussion 62–3.

McCarty, M. F. "Enhanced synovial production of hyaluronic acid may explain rapid clinical response to high-dose glucosamine in osteoarthritis." *Medical Hypotheses* June 1998;50(6):507–10.

"Monograph: Boswellia serrata." *Alternative Medicine Review* August 1998;3(4):306–7.

Moreno, B. "Treasures from the sea." *Better Nutrition* August 1999;39–41.

Pipitone, V. R. "Chondroprotection with chondroitin sulfate." *Drugs Under Experimental and Clinical Research* 1991;17(1):3–7.

Qiu, G. X., et al. "Efficacy and safety of glucosamine sulfate versus ibuprofen in patients with knee osteoarthritis." *Arzneimittelforschung* May 1998;48(5):469–74.

Safayhi, H., et al. "Boswellic acids: novel, specific, nonredox inhibitors of 5-lipoxygenase." *Journal of Pharmacology and Experimental Therapies* June 1992;261(3):1143–6.

Sander, O., G. Herborn, and R. Rau. "Is H15 (resin extract of Boswellia serrata, "incense") a useful supplement to established drug therapy of chronic polyarthritis? Results of a double-blind pilot study." *Z Rheumatol* February 1998;57(1):11–6.

Sandoval-Chacon, M., et al. "Antiinflammatory actions of cat's claw: the role of NF-kappaB." *Alimenary Pharmacology and Therapy* December 1998;12(12):1279–89.

Whitehouse, M. W., et al. "Anti-inflammatory activity of a lipid fraction (Lyprinol) from the NZ green-lipped mussel." *Inflammopharmacology* 1997;5:237–246.

Wilder, R. L. "Adrenal and gonadal steroid hormone deficiency in the pathogenesis of rheumatoid arthritis." *Journal of Rheumatology Supplement* March 1996;44:10–2.

Williams, C. A. "The flavonoids of Tanacetum parthenium and T. vulgare and their anti-inflammatory properties." *Phytochemistry* June 1999;51(3):417–23.

Williams, P. J., R. H. Jones, and T. W. Rademacher. "Reduction in the incidence and severity of collagen-induced arthritis in DBA/1 mice, using exogenous dehydroepiandrosterone." *Arthritis and Rheumatism* May 1997;40(5):907–11.

CHAPTER EIGHT

Astin, J. A. "Stress reduction through mindfulness meditation. Effects on psychological symptomatology, sense of control, and spiritual experiences." *Psychotherapy and Psychosomatics* 1997;66(2):97–106.

Batson, G. "Alleviating arthritis pain and discomfort: how the Alexander Technique can help." A Web page provided as a service by Alexander Technique Nebraska and the Ontario Centre for the Alexander Technique.

Belanger, A. Y. "Physiological evidence for an endogenous opiate-related pain-modulating system and its relevance to TENS. A review." *Physiotherapy Canada* 1985;37(3):163–168.

Berman, B. M., et al. "Efficacy of traditional Chinese acupuncture in the therapy of symptomatic knee osteoarthritis: a pilot study." *Osteoarthritis and Cartilage* June 1995;3(2):139–42.

Birch, S., et al. "Acupuncture in the therapy of pain." *Journal of Alternative and Complementary Medicine* Spring 1996;2(1):101–24.

Christensen, B. V., et al. "Acupuncture treatment of severe knee osteoarthrosis. A long-term study." *Acta Anaesthesiologica Scandinavia* August 1992;36(6):519–25.

Dolby, V. "Ouch! Nutritional approaches to help you say 'aaahh.'" *Better Nutrition* May 1998;18.

Domangue, B. B., et al. "Biochemical correlates of hypnoanalgesia in arthritic pain patients." *Journal of Clinical Psychiatry* June 1985;46(6):235–8.

Garfinkel, M. S. "Yoga-based intervention for carpal tunnel syndrome: a randomized trial." *JAMA* November 11, 1998;280(18):1601–3.

Garfinkel, M. S., et al. "Evaluation of a yoga-based regimen for treatment of osteoarthritis of the hands." *Journal of Rheumatology* December 21, 1994;(12):2341–3.

Guan, Z., and J. Zhang. "Effects of acupuncture on immunoglobulins in patients with asthma and rheumatoid arthritis." *Journal of Traditional Chinese Medicine* June 1995;15(2):102–5.

Haanen, H. C., et al. "Controlled trial of hypnotherapy in the treatment of refractory fibromyalgia." *Journal of Rheumatology* January 1991;18(1):72–5.

Horn, C. "13 Ways to Wipe Out Pain." *Natural Health,* January–February 1999:123–139.

Johnson, M. I., C. H. Ashton, and J. W. Thompson. "The clinical use of TENS." *Journal of Orthopedic Medicine* 1992;14(1):3–12.

Kabat-Zinn, J. "The clinical use of mindfulness meditation for the self-regulation of chronic pain." *Journal of Behavioral Medicine* June 1985;8(2):163–90.

———. "An outpatient program in behavioral medicine for chronic pain patients based on the practice of mindfulness meditation: theoretical considerations and preliminary results." *General Hospital Psychiatry* April 1982;4(1):33–47.

Liu, X., et al. "Effect of acupuncture and point-injection treatment on immunologic function in rheumatoid arthritis." *Journal of Traditional Chinese Medicine* September 1993;13(3):174–8.

Madrid, A. D., and S. H. Barnes. "A hypnotic protocol for eliciting physical changes through suggestions of biochemical responses." *American Journal of Clinical Hypnotism* October 1991;34(2):122–8.

Mills, W. W., and J. T. Farrow. "The transcendental meditation technique and acute experimental pain." *Psychosomatic Medicine* April 1981;43(2):157–64.

Nespor, K. "Pain management and yoga." *International Journal of Psychosomatics* 1991;38(1–4):76–81.

Starbuck, J. "Herbal pain relief: nature to the rescue." *Better Nutrition* May 1998;50–56.

Glossary

acetaminophen: A pain-relieving drug that works by blocking pain messages to the brain.

allopathic medicine: Conventional, drug- and surgery-based medicine; emphasis is on finding "magic bullets" to cure disease.

alternative medicine: Medical practices based on use of natural substances and non-invasive healing; approaches disease as a symptom of imbalance and seeks to correct it.

arachidonic acid: Scientific name for fats found in meats and dairy products; raw material for pro-inflammatory eicosanoids.

arthritis: Literally, inflammation of the joints; used in reference to over one hundred different diseases that strike connective tissues, causing joint pain, swelling, degeneration, and disability.

autoimmune disease: Where the immune system loses its ability to distinguish between "self" and "not-self," and attacks the body's tissues, causing inflammation.

bursae: Fluid-filled pads that provide cushioning between bones and between bones and skin.

candidiasis: Overgrowth of yeasts, or *candida,* which release toxins into the body and stimulate immune responses.

cartilage: Spongy, springy connective tissue that provides padding and lubrication between ends of bone.

chondroblasts: Cells in cartilage that make protein and carbohydrate substances that fill in the spaces in collagen.

chyme: Food that has been partially digested in the stomach.

collagen: Strong, ropelike strands of protein that form gridworks upon which connective tissues are built.

collagenases: Enzymes that digest collagen.

complementary medicine: The best of both medical worlds; use of allopathic and alternative medical practices in concert with one another.

corticosteroids: Synthetic versions of cortisol, a natural anti-inflammatory hormone; commonly taken in pill form for rheumatoid arthritis and injected into joints for osteoarthritis.

cortisol: An anti-inflammatory hormone; also known as a "stress hormone" because levels go up during times of stress.

cyclooxygenase (COX): A type of enzyme that transforms arachidonic acid and gamma-linoleic acid (GLA) into pro-inflammatory eicosanoids.

COX-1: A form of COX that protects the lining of the gastrointestinal tract; blocking it with NSAID drugs often leads to ulcers.

COX-2: A specific form of COX enzyme that increases inflammation.

delayed food allergy: The intestinal immune system becomes sensitized to a food, causing inflammation; this leads to the formation of tiny leaks in the intestinal wall, allowing incompletely digested food particles into the circulation; the immune system responds, causing allergic reactions that may be subtle or obvious.

DMARDs: Disease-modifying antirheumatic drugs; used to treat advanced rheumatoid arthritis; work by suppressing the immune system.

eicosanoids: Locally acting hormones that mediate inflammation, thickness of blood, and pain responses; include leukotrienes, prostaglandins, and thromboxanes.

Endorphins: The body's natural painkilling biochemicals.

fructooligosaccharides: Probiotic bacteria's favorite food.

glycosaminoglycans (GAGs): Sugar and protein molecules that link together to form proteoglycans; glucosamine sulfate is an example of a GAG.

H. pylori (helicobacter pylori): Bacteria responsible for many cases of ulcer, heartburn, and chronic indigestion.

hyaluronic acid: A substance in synovial fluid; gives fluid its viscosity and shock-absorbing quality.

hydrochloric acid: The strong acid made by the stomach for digestion.

inflammation: The body's immune response to injury, or to invasion by infectious agents or toxins; characterized by heat, swelling, redness, and pain; in osteoarthritis, there is rarely any inflammation, but it's the hallmark of rheumatoid arthritis and other autoimmune diseases.

isometric exercise: Working muscles against resistance that does not move; for example, pushing against an immovable object to exercise the arm muscles.

macronutrients: Carbohydrates, protein, and fats; the calorie-containing parts of the food we eat.

micronutrients: Vitamins, minerals, and other phytochemicals that have nutritional value but contain no calories.

NSAIDs: Non-steroidal anti-inflammatory drugs; first-line allopathic treatment for osteoarthritis and rheumatoid arthritis; work by affecting balance of eicosanoids.

omega-3 fats (eicosapentaenoic acid, or EPA): The type of fat found in fish, walnuts, and pumpkin seeds; can only be transformed into anti-inflammatory eicosanoids; flax contains alpha-linoleic acid, an omega-3 fat that is transformed into EPA in the body.

omega-6 fats (gamma-linoleic acid, or GLA): The type of fat found in vegetable, evening primrose, and soybean oils; there is some controversy about its use for rheumatoid arthritis, because it can be made into both pro- and anti-inflammatory eicosanoids.

orthomolecular medicine: The use of high doses of nutrients found in foods to treat illness.

pepsin: A protein-digesting enzyme.

probiotics: "Friendly" bacteria that live in the gastrointestinal, genital, and urinary tracts; manufacture vitamins and keep "unfriendly" bacteria and yeasts from becoming overgrown.

proteoglycans: Made of glycosaminoglycans (GAGs); weave through collagen fibers to form connective tissue.

putrefactive bacteria: "Bad" bacteria, such as e.coli and clostridium, that can become overgrown and toxic to the body if "good" bacterial populations decrease.

specificity: Describes the ability of a drug to affect one body process without affecting any others.

substance P: A biochemical that stimulates sensations of pain.

toxin: Any substance that can do damage to living tissue; *exotoxins* come into the body from outside, while *endotoxins* are formed within the body in the natural course of its day-to-day functions.

tumor necrosis factor: A cancer-fighting arm of the immune system, thought to be involved in the causes of both osteoarthritis and rheumatoid arthritis.

Index